90 SECONDS TO MUSCLE PAIN RELIEF

THE FOLD AND HOLD METHOD

BY DALE L. ANDERSON, M.D.

CompCare® Publishers

MINNEAPOLIS, MINNESOTA

©1992 by Dale L. Anderson, M.D.
All rights reserved.
Published in the United States
by CompCare Publishers

Reproduction in whole or part, in any form, including storage in a
memory device system, is forbidden without written permission
except that portions may be used in broadcast or printed commentary
or review when attributed fully to the author and publication by
names.

Library of Congress Cataloging-in-Publication Data
Anderson, Dale L. 1933–
    90 seconds to muscle pain relief / Dale L. Anderson.
       p. cm.
    ISBN 0-89638-242-7
    1. Myalgia—Treatment.   I. Title.
RC925.5.A52   1992   91-40444
616.7′4—dc20   CIP

Cover and interior design by MacLean and Tuminelly
Illustrations by Al Hage

Inquiries, orders, and catalog requests should be addressed to:
CompCare Publishers
2415 Annapolis Lane
Minneapolis, Minnesota 55441
Call 612-559-4800 or
toll free 1-800-328-3330

  6   5   4   3   2   1
 97   96   95   94   93   92

To my wife, Barbara, and our family.

Contents

Acknowledgments
Important note to readers

Chapter One: An Introduction to *Fold and Hold*   **1**

The child shall lead us   4
Rediscovering your physician within   6
What this book covers   7
What *Fold and Hold* is not   8
Who can use this book   9
Fold and Hold is safe   10
The healthy pleasures of touch   10
Approaching pain in a new way   11
How to use this book   12

Chapter Two: Principles of *Fold and Hold*   **13**

How *Fold and Hold* came about   14
Unlocking the mystery of muscle spasm   15
Empower yourself with *Fold and Hold*   16
Fold and Hold in four steps   17
Keys to the strategy of *Fold and Hold*   22
How pain occurs in daily life   22
    How muscles become weak and stiff   26
The role of Mother Nature   27
The virtues of self-reliance   29
Fold and Hold is not *the* answer   30
Listen to your body's signals   30

Chapter Three: Using *Fold and Hold* to Relieve Specific Areas of Pain

31

How this chapter is organized	31
Getting our terms straight	34
Working with your personal physician	35
Ankle pain	36
Back pain: Low back (iliopsoas muscle spasm)	38
Back pain: Low back/abdomen pain that feels better with sitting	43
Back pain: Low back/abdomen pain that feels better with standing	45
Back pain: Rotating-at-the-waist pain	48
Back pain: Tailbone (coccyx pain)	50
Back pain: Upper back	52
Buttocks/back tightness and pain (piriformis muscle spasm with or without sciatica)	55
Elbow pain: Golfer's elbow	59
Elbow pain: Tennis elbow	62
Foot pain: Bunion pain	65
Foot pain: Heel pain/spur (spasm of the flexor digitorum brevis)	66
Foot pain: Tenderness on the forefoot (metatarsalgia)	72
Hand pain: Weeder's thumb/Tea sipper's thumb	73
Head and neck pain	75
Fold and Hold for the upper neck: Using the de-tenniser	76
Assisted *Fold and Hold* for the upper neck	79
Fold and Hold for the rest of the neck	80
Hip pain (tensor fasciae latae muscle spasm)	82
Shin splints	84
Shoulder pain: "Pouring the coffee" pain (tendonitis biceps brachii)	87
Shoulder pain: "Putting on a coat" pain	89

Shoulder pain: "Raising the arm" pain   92
Wrist pain: Carpal tunnel syndrome   94

**Chapter Four: Common Questions
about *Fold and Hold***   **97**

**Chapter Five: Five More Keys
to Treating and Preventing Pain**   **103**

Stretching and strengthening muscles   104
     Using the relaxing stretch   105
Stretching scar tissue   106
Strengthening muscles   107
Maintaining a healthful sitting posture   108
Using a lumbar roll   110
Exercises to improve posture   112
Caring for your back   113
     Warning signs that your back needs attention   113
Why discs move around   114
A short history of back arching   116
The benefits of back arching   118
Get back your youthful back   119
A safe position for cooling down   121
Try this thirty-second back-arching exercise   122
Allowing yourself some pain   124
     Looking at your own experience of pain   125
Pain and the brain   126
Living with pain   127
Good pains and bad pains   127
More about bad pains   128
Using the pain scale   129
Healing the emotional side of pain   130

About the author   134
About the illustrations   134

Acknowledgments

A special thanks to:

The dedicated and professional staff at CompCare Publishers.

The 350 physician colleagues and the 2,000 support staff of Park Nicollet Medical Center in Minneapolis, Minnesota. Thanks for the professional medical environment that encourages physician individuality, innovation, and entrepreneurship. And thanks for the group's commitment to the highest medical standards and its constant striving to improve the delivery and quality of health care.

Jim Toscano, executive vice president, Park Nicollet Medical Foundation, for encouraging the writing of this book.

The platform friends of the National Speakers Association for setting high standards and inspiring me to strive to achieve their expected quality of excellence.

Lawrence H. Jones, D.O., author of *Strain and Counterstrain,* whose research on mobilization techniques deeply influenced my thinking about pain relief.

Philip E. Greenman, D.O., professor of biomechanics, College of Osteopathic Medicine, Michigan State University, and his associates who share and effectively teach the "Principles of Manual Medicine."

Harold R. Schwartz, D.O., of Columbus, Ohio, who is a master at teaching the "magic right moves" of Strain and Counterstrain.

John Pope for his promotional advice and counsel.

Douglas Toft for his editorial and writing expertise and talent.

Al Hage for his wonderful rendition of these illustrations.

Important note to readers

Although *Fold and Hold* is a safe way to relieve common muscular pain, the information in this book cannot take the place of personalized medical treatment. Check with your physician to treat any persistent ache or pain.

1 An Introduction to Fold and Hold

The young man was suffering so much from pain in his lower back that he could not stand erect. In fact, he had endured this discomfort for over four months, and treatment by two chiropractors had brought him no relief. During that time, the symptoms remained largely the same: pain and loss of sleep. While in bed, he would wake every fifteen minutes or so, struggle to find a position of comfort, and finally doze off again. All this was true even though the man had been in excellent shape, with the grace and power of an athlete.

This man's search for an answer to his condition brought him to an osteopath named Lawrence H. Jones. At first, Dr. Jones was stymied: eight weeks of his treatments resulted in no progress. Finally Jones decided to devote one session simply to helping his patient find a comfortable sleeping position. He helped the young man assume several postures, pausing to ask if any of them felt better than the others.

After twenty minutes of experimenting, they

succeeded in finding a position of surprising comfort. Though Jones suspected the benefit was temporary, it was literally the only sign of hope that any treatment had produced. He advised the young man to remain propped in the position for several minutes. That way, he could perhaps remember the position well enough to find it the next time he went to sleep. At this point, Jones left the room to attend to some other business. And the patient fell asleep.

When Jones returned some time later, he found the young man standing comfortably erect. "He was overjoyed and so was I," wrote Jones, "but more than that I was astonished. At that visit nothing had been done for the patient but positioning for comfort, and that had succeeded where my best efforts had failed repeatedly."

Jones discovered, completely by accident, one of the secrets of a technique he called *Strain and Counterstrain*. I've modified that technique and developed it into a treatment called *Fold and Hold*. This is a simple way to relieve pain in muscles and joints—easy enough to perform yourself, without drugs, surgery, or even a trip to the doctor's office.

I recommend *Fold and Hold* because it's worked for me in the day-to-day job of treating common aches. Like Dr. Jones, I can tell some stories about sudden relief from pain.

One of the more common pains I've worked with is buttock pain often diagnosed as sciatica. Arvid Johnson was a runner who often complained about tightness in his buttocks. Once, after a long car ride, he suddenly developed a severe worsening of the pain in the buttocks with pain radiating to the back, into the leg, and down to the foot. This pain was incapacitating and markedly altered his lifestyle. Not only was he unable to run, he frequently could not attend meetings and was often awakened at night with pain. Johnson sought help from chiropractors, physicians, and physical therapists. All their treatments and exercises proved ineffective.

Luckily, this man's CAT (computerized axial tomography) scan showed only a slightly bulging disc with no nerve root impingement. (A significant disc bulge is found normally in over 50 percent of our population. These disc bulges are often blamed for the pain—wrongly blamed, I might add.) As Dr. Jones did in treating the young man with low back pain, I helped Johnson find a position of comfort. In this case, it meant placing one of Johnson's legs in the "frog position"—turned out to the side, with the knees raised and bent. (See figure for *Fold and Hold* hip pain—piriformism, page 83.) Doing so relaxed a muscle called the piriformis, which was pinching on the sciatic nerves. In ninety seconds, the pain he had been experiencing for months was gone. If this diagnosis had been made on the first visit to a practitioner, many unnecessary expenses could have been avoided.

Another example is Mrs. Olson, who had spent the summer on a bus tour of Europe. During the trip, she developed a severe ache, pain, and tenderness over her outer hip. It hurt her to walk. It also hurt to lie in bed on her sore side, resulting in many sleepless nights. Sitting hurt, too, especially if she tried to cross the leg on the painful side of her body over her opposite leg. Her pain resulted from a spasm in a lateral hip muscle, the tensor fasciata—not from trochanteric bursitis, as it had been diagnosed.

Like the other people I've mentioned, this patient's story included a litany of ineffective treatments: physical therapy, new shoes, anti-inflammatory drugs, all to no avail. Even a cortisone steroid injection gave only temporary relief.

With *Fold and Hold*, the story changed. We treated the ache, pain, and tenderness over her outer hip by shortening this muscle. This was accomplished by helping her "fold" the body over her tender spot. For Mrs. Olson, this meant holding her leg in an outward and upward position for ninety seconds. (See the illustration for the *Fold and Hold* for hip pain, page 83.) This simple manipulation gave her complete relief.

The position she assumed in my office, though it looked awkward, was comfortable for her. I believe that Mother Nature was giving Mrs. Olson subtle cues to find this position on her own. If she had listened to those directions, and known the wisdom of *Fold and Hold*, she could have treated herself much sooner, avoiding many hours and dollars of medical expense.

These stories illustrate two fundamental facts about pain. First, many common muscular aches and pains persist, even with conventional drug treatments, surgery, and physical therapy. Moreover, these pains sometimes disappear spontaneously, as if by magic.

In essence, *Fold and Hold* aims to uncover the secrets of this "magic"—to help you make the right moves that result in pain relief.

What is *Fold and Hold*? In brief, it's a ninety-second self-treatment technique. *Fold and Hold* could help you relieve 75 percent of the common muscular aches and pains you experience. It's simple, once you master some basic concepts and a few of the magic "right moves." *Fold and Hold* works because it draws on the natural healing power of the body. When you apply this technique, you're merely cooperating with Mother Nature and unleashing the "physician within."

The child shall lead us

Remember when you were sick in bed as a child and Grandma asked, "How can I make you more comfortable?" She was getting at the essence of *Fold and Hold*: finding a comfortable position ("folding" the body to relieve pain) and holding that position. Pain relief often occurs when we get into comfortable positions during sleep. My own belief is that if people would allow themselves to sleep comfortably, many of their pains would go away. This is often hard for adults, because the comfortable position may be awkward or, worse yet, "indecent."

Children are natural masters of pain control. They have not developed many of the lifestyle habits and anxieties that promote pain in adults. They usually don't have the aches and pains adults complain about. Children keep their muscles flexible and loose. They spontaneously find their comfortable position during sleep—no matter how uncomfortable that position appears. Without realizing it, they naturally apply the basic principles and techniques of *Fold and Hold*.

Many adults who see a child sleeping in an awkward position will "straighten the child out"—especially those adults who've learned that there are "proper" positions to assume while sleeping. Unfortunately, this repositioning interrupts the natural pain treatment being provided by Mother Nature. Even worse, it teaches children that it is not acceptable to let themselves go into "crazy" positions.

Let's think this out a little further. Have you ever seen a young child wake up with pain? Probably not. Consider some further questions. Don't children usually move from one seemingly uncomfortable position to another during a nap or at night? Could part of the secret of a pain-free youth be sleeping in these "unnatural" positions? Is nature working a treatment for potential aches and pains as the child sleeps? Does our society tend to "grow into" more aches and pains as we get older because we come to comply more with how we *should* sleep than how the body *wants* to sleep? And should we not permit ourselves as adults to get into those strange positions, as we did in childhood?

Fold and Hold answers "yes" to these questions and prompts us to heed the advice of our "physician within."

Rediscovering your physician within

Through the years I studied mobilization techniques out of curiosity, as a kind of medical hobby. These techniques involve moving the body into various positions to relieve pain. After observing these "manmade" techniques and contrasting them with the mobilization techniques practiced by Mother Nature, one thing became clear: yes, the body often needs and wants mobilization. Yet the body has the capability to mobilize itself. And it can do so if we will only let ourselves go into a *comfortable* position. This is true no matter how awkward, how funny, how grotesque, or how strange that comfortable position may be. Let's combine *Strain and Counterstrain* and other osteopathic techniques *with* the gentle, caring, caressing, comforting mobilization we can do to ourselves with the assistance of Mother Nature. I call the result *Fold and Hold*.

You can regain your natural ability to feel, understand, and read your body. You can master methods of pain control by relearning the childlike, easy-to-understand, easy-to-apply techniques explained in this book. Again, the magic of pain control involves learning how to make the right moves. We can do this simply by listening to the body's "desire" for a position of comfort. Then we can assist nature by folding into that position and holding or resting in that comfortable treatment position for a minimum of ninety seconds.

This is a medically sound but nontechnical book, comprising the homespun ideas of a primary care physician. (I see myself as a primary care physician, even though much of my orthopedic medicine practice consists of seeing people referred to me by others.) I've enjoyed reading the body codes that unlock many secrets of pain relief. These techniques come not just from theory, but from observing how people experienced such relief—sometimes for no apparent reason. In thirty-five years of patient care I have seen many "miraculous" incidences of pain relief. Many times I have asked myself, WHY? Many of these answers, as I interpret them, are in this book.

What this book covers

This book has several aims:

- To acquaint you with the many factors that contribute to pain—factors you can control.
- To convince you that muscle spasm is one of the leading causes of body aches and pains.
- And, most important of all, to explain how you can erase many of these common aches and pains.

Throughout this book, we'll keep returning to the four basic steps of *Fold and Hold:*

1. Find a tender or painful spot on your body.
2. Fold your body over the tender spot until that spot disappears or becomes 75 percent improved and the painful condition is relieved.
3. Hold this comfortable treatment position for at least ninety seconds.
4. Return slowly to a normal position.

That's *Fold and Hold,* in a nutshell. Much of this book is devoted to explaining these four steps in more detail.

Chapter Two begins by explaining some of the basic concepts behind *Fold and Hold*. Understanding these can help you apply *Fold and Hold* more intelligently, with a greater understanding of what you are doing.

In Chapter Three you'll find step-by-step, illustrated instructions. There you'll see how to apply *Fold and Hold* to specific areas of the body.

Almost everyone has questions when they use *Fold and Hold* for the first time. Chapter Four answers some of the more common ones.

Beyond the four steps of *Fold and Hold*, there are several more things you can do to help Mother Nature relieve pain. They include stretching and strengthening the muscles, developing the habit of good posture, and caring for your back on a daily basis. Also important are learning the difference between "good pain" and "bad pain," as well as healing the emotional side of pain. These are strategies I recommend to nearly everyone as wise biomechanical maintenance for the body. Learn about them in Chapter Five.

What Fold and Hold is not

The biomechanical mobilization of *Fold and Hold* is not painful or forceful. It does not involve forcefully "cracking" and "popping" vertebrae and joints into place. Nor does it painfully stretch or apply pressure to muscles that are already strained. I believe that often such painful or forceful techniques give only temporary relief, which means they have to be given repeatedly. Often these procedures do little more than keep the patient "occupied" until nature "accidentally" cures the problem.

The "snap, crackle, pop" mobilization techniques can often give significant relief by "forcing" displaced tissue back into position. But the relief is usually short-lasting, and the displaced tissue will not "stay put." Why? Because the factors causing the malpositioning—the spastic muscles— are still present. In a short time, muscle spasm can reproduce the old malposition. This means the pain can recur.

I can agree that often certain tissue, like bone, can appear to be out of place. But often tissue is held out of place by tight muscles. Effective treatment means relaxing the muscles, allowing the malpositioned tissue to fall back into proper biomechanical alignment. Thus, cure can come with simple, comfortable, and natural relief of the tight muscles.

Fold and Hold is based on comfort—that is, relaxing the tight, spastic muscle, putting it to "sleep," and then waking it gently. After the restful sleep the muscle awakens to a "new day" and is ready to forget its unpleasant, painful past.

If you've had experience with yoga, *Fold and Hold* may seem familiar. In fact, yoga stretches approximate the comfortable position referred to in the second or "fold" step of *Fold and Hold*. Please note, however, that "yoga" here refers to the asanas, the physical stretches themselves, and not to any philosophy or religion.

Who can use this book

You do not need a medical background to use *Fold and Hold*. In fact, while writing this book I've assumed you have *no* medical training. At the same time, a secondary audience for this book includes physicians and other health practitioners: nurses, physical therapists, chiropractors, and massage therapists. These professionals can "prescribe" this book to people in pain as a way to supplement their treatments.

While I don't assume medical knowledge on your part, I do surmise that you've had certain attitudes about and experiences with bodily pain. For example, you've probably observed that pain often comes on with rapid movements that can suddenly send muscles into spasm. Say that you push a car out of snow or mud and the car suddenly lunges forward; you twist a tight jar cover and the cover suddenly releases; or you loosen a tight screw and the screwdriver suddenly slips. In each of these cases, the result can be a sudden spasm of muscles with accompanying pain. Usually the pain subsides in a short time, but too often it lingers for days, weeks, or months.

Perhaps you've also observed that pain sometimes goes away mysteriously—miraculously. Often this happens during the night, followed in the morning by pleasant relief from the acute or chronic pain. Why? Just keep reading. The answer becomes clear as we learn more about *Fold and Hold*.

One more note. *Fold and Hold* is a universal technique, effective for people of all ages, and for athletes in particular.

Fold and Hold is safe

Fold and Hold is based on the idea that you want to assume more responsibility for your health. As such, it's part of the growing movement toward medical self-care. You can apply *Fold and Hold* to yourself or to others to relieve pain, with or without a physician. Why do I believe in the safety of this technique, even when it's performed without a physician? For two reasons.

First, *Fold and Hold* means moving the body *slowly and gently*. In fact, this is how Mother Nature already treats you.

Second, it's safe because the body is moving *toward a position of comfort*. If at any time the person being treated starts complaining of more pain, tenderness, or unpleasant symptoms such as dizziness, then—whoa! We've overshot the position of comfort, or we are folding the body incorrectly.

Also understand that, while a majority of our pains are muscle-related, not all pains are muscular in origin. If your pain does not improve with the *Fold and Hold* method, or if it gets worse, by all means see your physician.

The healthy pleasures of touch

While you can do *Fold and Hold* alone, it's also true that other people can assist you, especially in finding and maintaining a comfortable position. Remember, the comfortable folded position may be awkward, and at times it may be easier to maintain that position with help.

One of the pleasures of applying *Fold and Hold* to friends and family members is drawing on the natural therapeutic power of touch. This power extends to the toucher as well as the person being touched.

Touching augments healing, in part because it can raise endorphin levels. Endorphins are powerful chemicals produced naturally in our bodies. Endorphin levels are raised by exercise, positive imaging, optimism, and healthy relationships. There's also evidence that the simple acts of smiling and laughing can raise endorphins. As natural opiates, endorphins have the power to block out pain and produce feelings of pleasure. In fact, they are anywhere from 200 to 2,000 times more powerful than injectable morphine. My first book, *J'ARM for the Health of It* (CompCare Publishers), examines endorphins in more detail.

Approaching pain in a new way

As you read this book, be prepared to rethink some of your ideas about pain. For example, many people believe that pain happens when a bone pinches tissues or a nerve, or when it rubs against another bone. In reality, pain is influenced and caused by a host of factors: muscle spasm, tissue toxins, tissue damage, inflammation, anxiety, family stress, beliefs, weather, allergies, and many more.

Yet muscle spasm is often the chief culprit in most of the pain I see, and it is significantly improved by relaxing muscles that are in spasm. Relieving the spasm by relaxing and then gently stretching these muscles is the essence of *Fold and Hold*. Other factors that aggravate and perpetuate the pain can be addressed more easily if we first master the pain-relieving technique of *Fold and Hold*.

How to use this book

In short, this is a medical self-help book that can stand alone or supplement medical treatment. Chapter Three is meant to be used for reference, like an encyclopedia. Don't feel you have to read it straight through.

Even more important, remember that the goal is not to memorize all the possible tender spots or each step of the instructions in Chapter Three. Think of the instructions as examples or illustrations of the four basic steps in *Fold and Hold*.

2 Principles of Fold and Hold

"Climbing stairs kills me!"

"I haven't been able to jog in months because of shooting pains in my leg."

"My tennis elbow is so painful I can't even lift my briefcase."

"My pain keeps me awake at night."

"My backache is a pain in the neck."

For years, I listened to these stories, frustrated because I was often unable to help. These complaints of unrelenting pain are the ones that leave physicians, as well as their patients, feeling helpless. Unless surgery is clearly indicated, there's often been little for the physician to do but prescribe medication, advise rest, and hope that with time, the curative power of the body will work its magic.

13

How Fold and Hold came about

I knew there must be something more we could do, so I began "exploring nonconventional treatment avenues"—I began studying what physicians call mobilization techniques. In brief, mobilization means helping the body find positions where it can move and function efficiently.

Many mobilization techniques are in use today. They are popular with several kinds of health providers, including physical therapists, osteopaths, chiropractors, and massage therapists. But in general, physicians have shied away from all this.

About twenty years ago, a friend who is an osteopathic physician convinced me of the benefits of mobilization. I took off the "mobilization blinders" that I was taught to wear during my medical training and started to study these techniques. This study was undertaken mainly at the Michigan State University School of Osteopathic Medicine, and with Dr. Harold R. Schwartz, an osteopath in Columbus, Ohio. Dr. Lawrence Jones, an osteopath and the developer of the *Strain and Counterstrain* method, was present at several of Dr. Schwartz's tutorial sessions.

Over the years these superb educational opportunities led to the perfecting of my own mobilization "moves." It has been very gratifying to observe the many therapeutic improvements that followed. I feel confident as a physician that these results, along with new scientific evidence backing them, will continue to convince more of my colleagues that some mobilization techniques are medically sound. We can incorporate them into conventional medical practice. Today many of my medical and osteopathic colleagues, as well as physical therapists, are learning and using these simple techniques. And they've helped teach many people how to reduce biomechanical pains—without drugs.

The goal of mobilization is to remold and reposition

the body in a way that restores normal body function and movement, thereby relieving pain. This same goal is shared by the mobilization theories of High Velocity/Thrust, Muscle Energy, Myofascial Release, Cranio Sacral Manipulation, and *Strain and Counterstrain*. Each theory, however, comes with its own set of complicated principles. These principles are sound. Yet they often involve scientific language that makes them difficult for fellow physicians to learn—and almost impossible for patients to master.

After studying and evaluating these theories, I came to some basic conclusions. First, through applying mobilization techniques, we can learn how to help people relieve pain. Just as nature can manipulate many of our aches and pains away, so can we. And nearly everyone, regardless of their medical understanding, can learn these techniques. Helping people understand these moves means explaining them in simple terms. That explanation is what you're holding in your hands right now.

"Modeling" is something you might do if you were posing for an artist painting your portrait. The painter might ask you to assume one position, stay there for a minute or two, then try another pose. After several tries, you'd find a stance that feels just right for the picture, and you'd hold that position. Finding the pose that works—mobilizing into the best position—is the essence of being a successful model. Mobilization, as practiced in *Fold and Hold*, is much like this. As the artist says in the artistic painting session, Mother Nature will say in the *Fold and Hold* session, "That's it! That's it! Hold it!"

Unlocking the mystery of muscle spasm

We've all had muscle spasms before. What most of us don't

realize is that our muscles are complicated. Muscles can be large or tiny, long or short. Frequently they are interlaced among many other muscles. Often it's difficult to know just where the spastic muscle is located. Most of the time this muscle is near the site of pain, but at times it can be some distance away.

A whole muscle or a small portion of a muscle can go into a spasm. Yet we aren't always going to recognize the source of pain as a muscle spasm. Instead we may experience it as pain without a source that we can identify.

Fold and Hold assumes that the pain we are feeling is caused by a muscle in spasm. This spasm is often identified as a very tender spot. Finding that spot may require some searching, and sometimes we just cannot locate it. Even in the latter case, however, we can still apply *Fold and Hold*.

Empower yourself with Fold and Hold

Using *Fold and Hold*, people have experienced drug-free relief from common, sometimes excruciating, pains. When they have a muscular pain that is modified (made either better or worse) with movement, they can try to treat themselves before seeking medical attention. This self-mobilization often makes any further treatment unnecessary.

I tell each of my patients that I will see them only three times. If by the third visit they feel no better, then mobilization will not be effective. If they do feel better, then they've learned how to perform the right moves on their own, without my assistance.

Recently a young varsity basketball player came into my office. This man could barely walk because the pain in his back/flank was so great. In addition, he could not pivot to pass the ball or go up for a rebound because of pain in his lower back. After one session of *Fold and Hold*, he was smiling and ready to play basketball again. He learned how his muscle spasm occurred and how to treat it himself if it recurs. (See back/flank pain, quadratus lumborum muscle, page 48.)

Some people have been so surprised at the relief *Fold and Hold* brings that they tell friends and relatives. One patient, a runner, has treated practically everyone in his health club with *Fold and Hold* or taught them to use it.

Even the editor of this book was helped by *Fold and Hold*. Early in the project, I discovered she was experiencing neck pain. Just by talking her through the *Fold and Hold* procedures over the phone, we were able to treat the pain successfully. Perhaps it was this fortuitous coincidence that made CompCare Publishers agree to develop this book. (In this case, a pain in someone else's neck led me to complete relief!)

Fold and Hold is a simple technique—so simple, in fact, that it's hard for most people to believe that it can work. Yet the simplicity of *Fold and Hold* does not detract from its power. I've seen people who have endured the same muscle pain for ten years experience permanent relief after one session of *Fold and Hold*.

Fold and Hold in four steps

Step One: Find the tender spot

Fold and Hold starts from one basic idea: For most aches and pains we will usually find a small area of the body that feels *very tender*. When you touch this area, the person in pain may jump and say, "Ouch! It *really* hurts there!" When that happens, you know you've found the eye of the hurricane, so to speak; the "epicenter" of the pain. I call this the *tender spot* or *zinger*.

Before you can *Fold and Hold*, you need to locate this tender spot. Most often it is a small, focal area of spasm in a muscle. It can also be a strain at the site where a spastic muscle attaches to a bone. Or, it can be a strain on tissues (such as ligaments or fascia) that are being stretched.

About 90 percent of the time, the muscle in spasm and its tender spot will be in or near the area of discomfort. Occasionally—in about 10 percent of pains—the spastic muscle and its tender spot will be on the opposite side of the body from where one experiences pain. (This occurs most often in back and neck pains.) In these rare cases, you may fold away from the tender spot instead of over the tender spot (see step 2).

Keep in mind, too, that there might be several tender spots, not just one. Perhaps more than one muscle is in spasm. This could account for residual pain you feel after an initial *Fold and Hold*.

Even when there are groups of muscles in spasm, *Fold and Hold* focuses on one spastic muscle at a time—the "mother muscle," which is the muscle having the tenderest spot. Our aim is to relieve the tender spot in this dominant muscle. Doing so can frequently relieve other tender spots as well. To use a homespun analogy from my own rural background: the mother muscle is the hen, and the other tender spots are chicks that follow her. In the same way, if you relieve the tender spot in the mother muscle, relief of other tender spots will follow.

Step Two: Fold the body over the tender spot (Find the comfortable position)

We can get our muscles out of spasm by shortening and relaxing them as much as possible. This is done when you fold over a tender spot until the pain goes away. When the tenderness goes away, we have put the spastic muscle to "sleep" in a shortened, relaxed, comfortable position. See Diagram 1.

The comfortable position is the "sweet spot"—the position where you experience pain relief. Finding it is a process of fine tuning, like tuning a guitar string or finding the combination that opens a safe.

To arrive at the sweet spot, monitor the tender spot. You can do this by applying slight pressure to the tenderness and folding until the tender spot *maximally* improves. If you're moving in the correct direction, you'll feel less tenderness and more general comfort. Move the wrong way, and you'll feel more tenderness and discomfort.

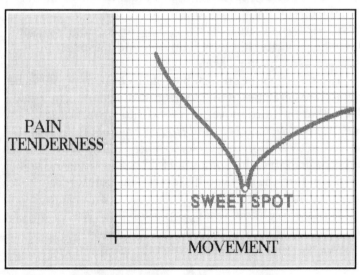

Diagram 1   In the fold—position of comfort.

Sometimes you may experience a move toward improvement, followed by a worsening of the pain. If that happens, you've overshot the comfortable position and you need to back up a bit. I call this *fine tuning*. By fine tuning, you can find the sweet spot.

Here it helps to learn the difference between passive and active pain. Active pain comes from working the spastic muscle; this is pain that comes when you load or activate the muscle. Passive pain comes when the muscle is stretched by an outside force, such as gravity or an opposing muscle pull from the opposite side of the body or limb. Active pain comes when working a muscle. The direction of active pain movement for a muscle is in the mirror-image opposite direction of the movement that elicits passive stretching pain of that muscle.

When performing *Fold and Hold*, the comfortable treatment fold will be toward the direction that causes active pain. The comfortable, treatment fold will be away from the direction that provokes passive stretching pain. Confused? Don't worry! Studying diagrams 2 and 3 on page 24 will help clarify this, as will understanding some of the treatments in Chapter Three.

In finding your comfortable fold treatment position, be prepared to get in poses that look quite awkward. The Bible tells us that the Lord moves in mysterious ways. So, at times, do people who *Fold and Hold*. Remember, if you find yourself in a position that looks strange, funny, or awkward but is comfortable, then *that's it*. Hold it. The way you look doesn't matter: the way you feel does. This comfortable fold is the treatment position.

Don't worry about what people will think if they walk into the room when you're in a comfortable position, however crazy it appears. The only relevant question is this: Does the tenderness lessen or go away in this position? Are you more comfortable? If your answer is yes, you're on the right track. Hold it!

Step Three: Hold the comfortable position for ninety seconds

The aim in this step is to let your body treat itself. The comfortable fold position is the treatment position, and the hold is the actual treatment. So be sure to hold for at least ninety seconds. If you like, hold the position longer than ninety seconds. The ninety-second figure is a minimum, not a maximum.

You may want to continue to touch the tender spot even after it becomes non-tender in order to sense the "release" of the muscle spasm. As you continue to apply light pressure for ninety seconds, you'll often find that the spastic muscle will relax, "melting" like butter. This can be a dramatic sensation.

Step four: Return to "normal position" SLOWLY

Again, holding the comfortable position means letting the muscle "sleep" for ninety seconds. During that time, the muscle "forgets" that it was in spasm. Moreover, it won't go back into spasm again, provided it is "awakened" very slowly—that is, if you take the time to gently move out of the folded position.

This step, even though it sounds simple and obvious, is crucial to the success of *Fold and Hold*. Even if you perform the first three steps effectively, you can lose what you've gained by getting out of your comfortable position too rapidly. Rapid movement can excite the waking muscle and provoke it to spasm again.

We can put it another way, comparing the muscle in spasm to a tired, irritable child. By holding your comfortable position, you're letting that child (muscle) take a short nap. Most children will react crossly if you awaken them too abruptly. In the same way, you can irritate a muscle or tissue by "awakening" it too fast—that is, by releasing your comfortable *Fold and Hold* position quickly. Treat the spastic muscle or strained tissue as gently as you'd wake an infant from a nap. You, too, deserve some tender, loving care.

Keys to the strategy of Fold and Hold

Most people feel significant relief after treatment with most mobilization and physical therapy techniques. Regrettably, however, it's common for the relief to last only for a matter of hours. Then the pain returns. This often happens when such techniques don't truly relax the spastic muscle. Instead of addressing the cause of the pain—the spastic muscle—they often only treat apparent body malpositions. Moreover, too often mobilization practitioners and therapists concentrate on physical symptoms and ignore psychological stress factors that get us "up tight." Instead of helping the spastic muscle to relax totally, they allow only partial relaxation. So the first key strategy of *Fold and Hold* is deep relaxation.

Another key is finding a treatment that relieves pain—specifically *for you*. That last phrase is important: The comfortable position or treatment that works for someone else is not necessarily the one that will work for you. *Fold and Hold* is based on the idea that each person is "one of a kind." And since the way people "store" pain is unique, effective treatment must take that uniqueness into account.

How pain occurs in daily life

The rough and tumble of daily life provides plenty of opportunities for muscle spasms to occur. Spasms happen with a single, sudden, large movement; through repetitive sudden, small, movements; and as a consequence of muscle bruises and tears.

Examples are easy to find. Take the person who falls asleep in an easy chair while reading, letting her head tip to one side. After twenty minutes in this position, she snaps to attention when the phone rings. Instantly, she feels pain stinging through her neck and shoulders.

Another example is the good Samaritan who comes upon a car stuck in mud or snow. Dutifully, he decides to help. Placing his full weight on his arms, our hero pushes against the rear bumper while the driver rocks the car back and forth, back and forth. Suddenly and without warning, the car frees itself and lurches forward. As our unfortunate victim stumbles to recover, several muscles may go into spasm.

Because such situations are so "everyday," we tend to overlook some of the common injury stresses to which we subject our muscles. These two examples are typical of a common cause of muscle spasm: quickly lengthening a shortened relaxed or a reflexly relaxed muscle. When that happens, we create a prime opportunity for muscle spasm.

Before going further, take a few minutes to look at Diagram 2 and Diagram 3 below. You may want to refer back to these diagrams when you try *Fold and Hold*.

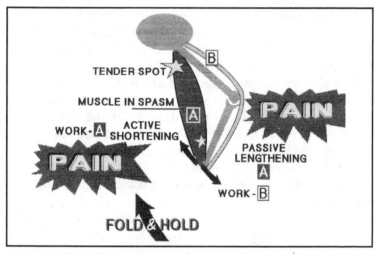

Diagram 2

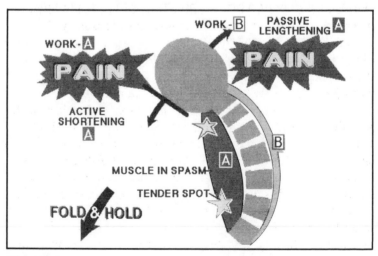

Diagram 3

Diagram 2 represents a hinged joint. This could be a hand, elbow, shoulder, hip, knee, ankle, foot, or toe. Diagram 3 represents any portion of the spine. There is no front or back, up or down, right or left to these diagrams. You could say these diagrams are generic. Muscle A is the muscle in spasm—shortened and containing tender spot(s). Muscle B is on the opposite side of the body or limb and when used has an action opposite to that of Muscle A. Muscle A is the muscle in spasm. Muscle A is the muscle to be treated by *Fold and Hold*.

The discomfort in irritable, spastic Muscle A can be provoked or worsened in three ways:

- Touching the tender spots
- Working or loading the muscle (active pain)
- Pulling or lengthening the muscle (passive pain)

The tender spots in these diagrams are denoted by stars. The movements that provoke pain are shown by arrows entitled A-active (shortening) and A-passive (lengthening).

Muscle B is on the opposite side of the joint or on the opposite side of the body from Muscle A. It has an action opposite to Muscle A. If and when Muscle B works and shortens, it causes a passive pull and lengthening of Muscle A. This passive lengthening causes pain in Muscle A.

Diagrams 1 and 2 show with a bold arrow the direction of the *Fold and Hold* treatment. Here Muscle A is "showing the way" to pain relief with *Fold and Hold*. Toward active work pain and away from passive stretch pain.

The fold of *Fold and Hold* gently assists irritable Muscle A to shorten and relax, moving it to a position of comfort which significantly reduces its tightness and its tender spot(s). Note that the direction for *Fold and Hold* relaxation treatment of Muscle A, the direction that permits a restful shortening of Muscle A, is in the same direction that causes pain with work or loading of Muscle A (active shortening). In addition, the *Fold and Hold* treatment position (bold arrow) is in the opposite direction of the passive movement that causes pull or lengthening of Muscle A.

In *Fold and Hold*, Muscle A is permitted to "go to sleep"—fold—for ninety seconds and then awakened slowly. This muscle wakes to a "new day" with no memory of its unpleasant past, ready to be stretched and strengthened by new life challenges.

How muscles become weak and stiff

If the spasm and discomfort of Muscle A has been chronic (of relatively long standing), then we will see both Muscles A and B become weakened. Muscle A will be weak because it cannot be worked without causing pain. Consequently, we work it less and less. And Muscle B is weakened because it has become loose and lengthened from disuse. If Muscle B attempts to work, its shortening results in a passive pull and pain of irritable Muscle A. Consequently, Muscle B also stops working and gets weaker and weaker. The longer the pain condition persists, the weaker both muscles become.

Spasm of a muscle results in the muscle being shortened. With chronic muscle spasm of Muscle A, the shortening can begin to "set." The individual muscle cells and surrounding connective tissue of Muscle A begin to stiffen into a contracted state.

After successful treatment with *Fold and Hold*, the tight, shortened (but no longer painful) muscle needs to be stretched, lengthened, and strengthened to regain its normal structure and functioning. Doing so helps it regain normal biomechanical function. The stretch needed is in the mirror-image opposite direction of the fold treatment position. If the fold is to bend forward, the stretch will be to bend backward. See Diagram 4.

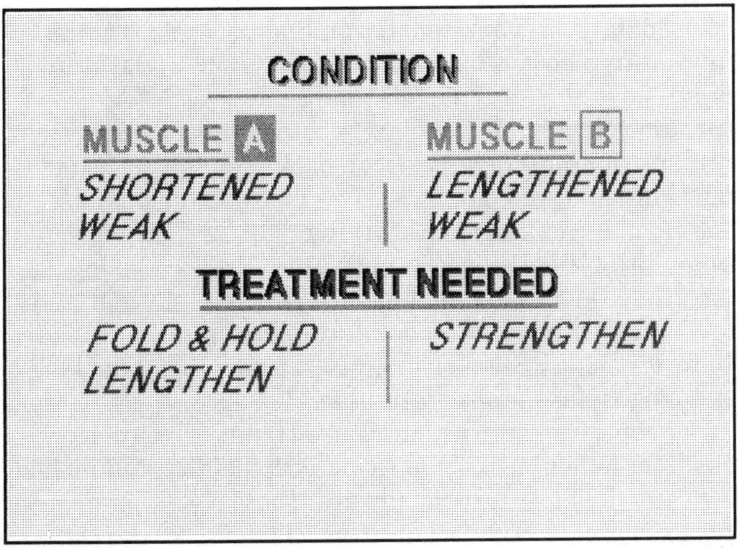

```
                    CONDITION

  MUSCLE  A               MUSCLE  B
  SHORTENED               LENGTHENED
  WEAK                    WEAK

           TREATMENT NEEDED

  FOLD & HOLD             STRENGTHEN
  LENGTHEN
```

Diagram 4

The role of Mother Nature

When you are in pain, as mentioned earlier, Mother Nature is prompting you to find a comfortable position. In fact, if *Fold and Hold* is effective, the treatment is done by nature and aided by the "physician within."

When people who are in pain come to see me, the first questions I ask are: What do you do that feels good? What activities do you like to do? What is your comfortable sitting, lying, or sleeping position? Whatever it is, I say: If it feels good, do more of it. For instance, many will say that they feel better when they get up and walk or become active. If so, they should walk more.

If an activity does not hurt while you are doing it, then the body's message is clear: do that activity more. If people feel some related pain the next day, this is because they're deconditioned in general and need to go into "training."

So the goal is to listen to your body, especially at the times your pain gets better or goes away. One of the most universal examples is the "end of the day stretch." After spending eight hours hunched over a desk, the natural response for most of us is to lean back in our chairs, extend our arms, and arch our backs. This is a spontaneous *Fold and Hold*. By arching we are in effect "folding" the body into a comfortable position. Mother Nature is always giving us directions on how to fold. When we hurt, we may naturally fold ourselves in our most comfortable position. Unfortunately, we don't usually go far enough or hold long enough to relax the spastic muscle.

People walk into my office in all kinds of weird positions—their necks bent to the side, their backs hunched forward, their legs turned outward. These positions are my key to where the body "wants to go." For people who are bent over in pain, the treatment isn't to straighten them up; when they stand straight, they will have greater pain. Remember that the concept behind *Fold and Hold* is to put yourself into a position of greatest comfort. If bending forward is more comfortable than standing up straight, then fold even farther forward and hold this position. Exaggerating the fold can be one way to control the "volume" of Mother Nature's message.

Always remember that the way to fold is in the opposite direction of the resting, stretched, passive position that produces more pain. For example, if your wrist hurts when passively bent upwards, then fold it down (toward the palm) for the treatment. Fold in the opposite direction from the passive lengthening-induced pain, and monitor the tender spot to find the precise position of muscle relaxation.

Throughout this book, I will be giving you instructions for finding positions to help remove certain pains. But all of these instructions are just guidelines. *The key to this entire book is finding the position where the tender spot goes away and you feel comfortable.*

Often it helps, if at all possible, to remember how you got your pain. Again, pains occur when you move abruptly from a position where a muscle is relaxed (either through shortening or by reflex) to a position where the muscle suddenly lengthens and consequently spasms. Often folding back into the position you were in before the sudden movement will help get rid of the pain.

So when you use *Fold and Hold*, be open to nature's suggestions: Follow your own body as it seeks a comfortable position.

The virtues of self-reliance

Self-reliance is the opposite of depending on a health professional to "fix" your pain and or of submitting yourself to long-term and expensive treatments. Of course, asking someone to occasionally teach and assist you with *Fold and Hold* is not the same as looking to them for a repeated "fix." Assistance is one thing; dependence is another.

One important point: though *Fold and Hold* incorporates some practices that are not in widespread use by physicians, it is not "anti-doctor." In fact, physicians can prescribe *Fold and Hold* as part of a total treatment program that may include physical therapy, drugs, or surgery. Physicians and chiropractors may wish to teach *Fold and Hold* to reduce their patients' dependence on being "fixed" and "adjusted." This encourages people to learn more about the biomechanics and their muscular pains and become actively involved in the solution.

Fold and Hold is not always *the* answer

Fold and Hold is meant to relieve many muscular pains relatively quickly—for example, after three sessions of finding a comfortable position. If *Fold and Hold* is not working at that point, other treatment may be called for.

Other factors can cause pain—for example, arthritis, fractures, malignancy, infections, emotional stress, etc. These call for treatment in addition to, or instead of, *Fold and Hold*. *Fold and Hold* is not a panacea but an adjunct technique. It can be used along with heat, massage, ice, and other treatments.

If you want to benefit fully from *Fold and Hold*, then remember one thing above all: don't just take my word for it. Don't believe any of it or take it on faith alone. Instead, use it. Experiment with it. Try *Fold and Hold* and see what works for you.

Listen to your body's signals

When applying *Fold and Hold*, don't do anything that causes a sharp pain (over 3 on a scale of 10). Your pain should not get worse as you do this technique. If it does, then stop. If you suspect that you have circulatory problems, proceed with caution when applying *Fold and Hold*. In particular, if you feel dizzy when arching your neck, then return to a normal position.

In short, *Fold and Hold* treatment is always to go to the most comfortable position. Used correctly, *Fold and Hold* will ease or eliminate many pains. If you encounter more discomfort, then you are folding in the wrong way, or the pain is caused by factors other than muscle spasm. In that case, see a physician.

3 Using Fold and Hold to Relieve Specific Areas of Pain

This chapter explains some of the more common muscle spasms. It must be emphasized, however, that there are many variations of single or related muscle group spasms. They may not follow the exact description of relief given here.

Yet the *Fold and Hold* principles are always the same: Fold for a comfortable position where the pain and the tender spot are relieved. Once you're in that position, hold for ninety seconds. Then slowly return to a more normal position.

How this chapter is organized

This chapter is organized like a mini-encyclopedia of common pains you can treat with *Fold and Hold*. You'll find entries, arranged alphabetically, for ankle pain, back pain, foot pain, hip pain, and more. Under each entry, you'll find four types of information:

1. Possible causes: These include the movements that could cause a muscle to go into spasm. There are three different types of provoking movements:

   ■ The first is rapid movement from a relaxed position. In the relaxed position, the involved muscle is shortened. The more the muscle is shortened, the more relaxed it becomes. With rapid movement the muscle is suddenly lengthened, leading to a spasm. This often happens when people awake from sleep suddenly, or when they move rapidly from a resting position.

   ■ A second kind of rapid movement takes place when a muscle is suddenly stretched from a reflex relaxation. This kind of relaxation takes place in a muscle whenever its opposing muscle is activated. For example, when you bend your arm at the elbow, the muscles on the front of the arm that flex your elbow (such as the biceps) are at work. However, the opposite muscles—those on the back of the arm that extend your elbow (such as the triceps)—are relaxed. These latter muscles are said to be reflexly relaxed.

   The harder a muscle works, the more the opposite muscle relaxes. What happens if you suddenly reduce the load on the working muscle— for example, if you're lifting a heavy object and it suddenly falls out of your hands? Then the working muscle quickly shortens and the opposite muscle (which was relaxed) quickly lengthens. This quick lengthening can result in a spasm in the reflexly relaxed muscle.

   ■ Repetitive loading of the muscle. For example, with the palm down, repeatedly lifting the wrist in picking up an object could result in spasm of the extensor muscles of the forearm. (See the instructions for "tennis elbow" on page 64.) Or, repeatedly pushing the wrist downward may result in spasm of the flexor muscles of the forearm. (Refer to carpal tunnel syndrome, page 94, and golfer's elbow, page 59.)

For several of the pains discussed in this chapter, I identify the muscle which I interpret to be in spasm, along with the function of that muscle. *It is not necessary for you to memorize the names, locations, or functions of these muscles.* This information is included for health professionals and for others who are interested. What's most crucial for you is this: Understand the location of the tender spots and how to apply *Fold and Hold* in each particular case.

2. *Symptoms:* Pain manifests itself in different ways for each of us. Keep in mind that we often feel or aggravate muscle pain in three different ways: when we apply pressure to a tender spot in an irritable, spastic muscle (such as by lying or sitting on it); when we work (load) an irritable muscle in spasm; or when we passively stretch an irritable muscle in spasm. (See Diagrams 2 and 3 on page 24.)

3. *Find the tender spot:* Here you'll find short instructions and an illustration that suggests where to look for tender spots. On the illustrations, each dot represents a potential tender spot. Usually these spots are located somewhere on the muscle in spasm. Remember, though, that these instructions are general guidelines. You might find a tender spot in locations other than those illustrated. Let your *body* be your guide. And let your fingers "do the walking" to find these "zingers."

4. *Fold and Hold*: The fold is the comfortable position, the one you assume to relax the spastic muscle and alleviate pain. HOLD this position for at least ninety seconds, and be sure to come out of this position slowly. Understanding the basics of the A and B muscle diagram on page 24 will help you find the most comfortable position, which is your fold position. You will fold toward the position that gives active pain—the opposite (mirror image) of the position that produces the passive, stretch discomfort.

Properly done, *Fold and Hold* is not painful. Remember that *Fold and Hold* is based on relaxing the muscles, not on applying pressure to the tender spot. You can, however, keep applying some pressure to the tender spot even after it has been relieved. The tender spot can often be felt as a thickening in the muscle—a "knot." Usually you'll be able to feel the knot "melt" as the muscle relaxes.

In Chapter Five you'll find instructions for stretching the spastic muscle and strengthening muscles to prevent pain from recurring.

Getting our terms straight

The instructions in this chapter use certain terms repeatedly. These will be more clear if you keep in mind the following definitions:

Front (anterior) and back (posterior) or forward and backward. Most of the time you can rely on common sense to tell you what the front and back sides of the body are. Possible exceptions are the arm and hands. When you stand, your knuckles and nails are on the back of the hand, and the palm is the front of the hand. The thumbs are pointing outward. Health practitioners use the term anterior for the front of the body and posterior for the back.

Up or down. Movement toward the head is up. Down is toward the feet.

Twist inward or outward or twist right or left. The arms and the legs can twist on a central longitudinal (up and down) axis. When you twist your arm, the thumb either moves inward (toward the center of the body) or outward (away from the center of the body). Likewise, when you twist your leg, the big toe either moves inward or outward.

Your torso, head, and neck also move on a central, longitudinal axis. The spine can twist to the right or left on this axis. Twisting your head to the right, for example, means your face will be turned to the right.

Bend. This term indicates movements that move the torso or head toward the side, front, or back. For instance, bending your head or the back to the right results in moving your right ear toward your feet. Bending the spine backwards is called *arching*.

Abduction, or outward. Refers to moving an arm or leg in a sideward direction away from the center of the body.

Adduction, or inward. Refers to moving the arm or leg toward the center of the body. Your arms and legs are alternately abducted and adducted when you do the common exercise known as "jumping jacks."

Flexion and extension. These terms describe movement around a joint. Flexing a joint makes the joint angle smaller (acute). Extension is moving the joint toward being straight. A few joints can move beyond straight and into a hyperextended position. These include the toes, ankle, knuckles, and wrist. For example, flexing the leg at the hip means bringing the knee to the chest; extending the leg means straightening it; and hyperextending the leg means bringing it backwards behind the body. Walking includes all these actions.

Right, left. When studying or following the instructions given in this chapter, keep in mind that the muscle spasms described are on the right side of the body. To perform *Fold and Hold* for a muscle on the left side, perform the corresponding movements toward the left.

Working with your personal physician

The instructions in this chapter represent my current views on treating the common aches and pains described. As I keep working with *Fold and Hold*, I continually change and refine these views. We in medicine have had good reason to change many of the beliefs we once regarded as fact. Twenty-five years ago, for instance, I told people not to eat fiber and not to arch their backs. Today back arching is "in," and if I had a good recipe for sawdust muffins I would pass it on to you.

What if your doctor disagrees with any of the advice I give in this book? Whose instructions do you follow? My answer is brief: You know your doctor, and your doctor knows you. *Follow the advice of your personal physician.*

Ankle pain

Possible causes

One of the most common traumatic injuries I see in the emergency department or in the orthopedic medicine clinic is the sprained ankle. When the foot is accidentally twisted inward and the ankle rolls outward, some of the ligaments over the outer ankle can be partially or completely torn. With proper care these ligaments will usually heal, and the ankle should become pain-free in a few weeks.

Sometimes a pain over the outer ankle persists for months, however. This may be due to a spasm in the peroneous longus muscle. This is a long muscle that arises on the upper, outer side of the lower leg. It has a long tendon that passes behind the outer bony prominence of the ankle (the lateral malleolus) and attaches to the under, inner side of the foot near the arch.

The action of this muscle is to twist and bend the foot and ankle outward (opposite the direction they move in an ankle sprain). At the time of the ankle sprain, this muscle is suddenly lengthened and it may go into spasm.

Symptoms

Symptoms of ankle pain include tenderness and pain over the outer ankle after the ankle is sprained. At first, the pain is usually due to injury of the ligaments. But if the pain persists, then it is likely that the peroneous longus muscle is in chronic spasm.

People with this condition find walking painful. And the better the shoe and arch support, the worse the resulting discomfort. Often these people walk better with sandals, in flats without arch supports, or in bare feet.

Twisting and bending the foot and ankle to simulate the original injury passively stretches the irritable peroneous longus muscle. This aggravates the pain. When the muscle is worked by pushing an object out to the side with the forefoot, this discomfort can also be aggravated.

Find the tender spot

The tender spot is often near the outer bony prominence (lateral malleolus) of the ankle. This spot can also be in the "belly" of the muscle, higher up the outer side of the lower leg.

Fold and Hold

The fold position will be the mirror image—that is, the opposite—of the position where the sprain occurred. Pain in the tender spot will lessen as you: (1) bend the foot outward at the ankle, (2) position the foot or ankle downward in the direction of the sole, and (3) twist the foot slightly outward. Imagine that you're folding over the tender spot. While you're sitting in a chair, you can place the inside of the foot on the floor with the ankle rolled outward. The hand touching the tender spot can exert some downward pressure to increase the fold, if needed, to relieve spot tenderness. *Fold and Hold* for at least ninety seconds and release slowly.

When you're done, stretch slowly and gently in the opposite direction from the fold. This stretch simulates the position in which the sprained ankle occurred.

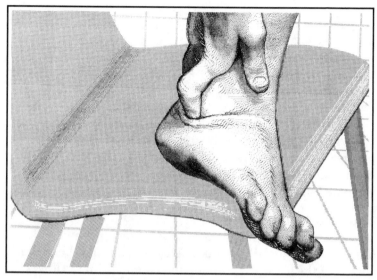

Figure 1   *Fold and Hold* for ankle pain.

Back pain: Low back
(iliopsoas muscle spasm)

Possible causes

Two muscles unite to form the iliopsoas. These muscles originate on the front of the back wall of the pelvic bone, and on the front of the lower vertebrae of the back. The iliopsoas tendon attaches in the groin area to the upper, inner part of the large bone (femur) in the upper leg. The action of this muscle is to flex the thigh at the hip, bringing the thigh and knee up to the abdomen and chest.

I commonly see this kind of low back pain in people who kneel on one knee for a prolonged period of time. This often takes place while they're gardening or doing a project on the floor. Such activity forces them to bend over and kneel. If they kneel on the left knee, the right thigh and knee are positioned near the chest. The right iliopsoas muscle is maximally shortened, in a relaxed position. If this position

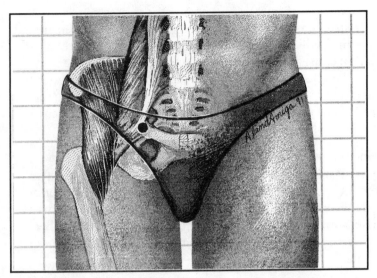

Figure 2   Location of the iliopsoas muscle and tender spot.

is maintained, the muscle may "go to sleep." (See Figure 6, kneeling treatment position.)

What happens when the telephone rings or someone asks them to hurry back to the house from the garden? Usually these people stand up quickly from the bending, kneeling position. When this happens, the relaxed right iliopsoas muscle is startled. It "panics" and reacts by going into spasm.

The iliopsoas muscle can also be deeply relaxed when you sit with one knee tucked up and held under the chin. This is a fairly common position for watching television. This muscle can go into spasm if you suddenly rise from this position. (See Figure 4, sitting treatment position.)

Symptoms

Standing up straight hurts because this action stretches the spastic muscle. Pain is often experienced in the back, since this is where the muscle originates. Bending to the opposite side stretches the muscle and aggravates the pain. Lifting the thigh when walking up stairs also causes pain; this action causes the spastic muscle to work.

People with this pain often report that it feels better to sit than to stand. They may feel better yet if they bring the right knee up closer to the chest. It simply hurts to be in any position other than bending slightly forward.

Find the tender spot

It is often difficult to touch the tender spot for this pain. A tender spot, if you can find it, is commonly located over or on the outer prominence of the pubic bone. This spot may also be in the groin or the lower abdominal muscles; check this area, too. (See Figure 2, location of muscle and tender spots.)

Fold and Hold

As in most of the *Fold and Hold* treatments, finding the comfortable position and erasing the tender spot means getting back into a certain position: the position you were in prior to the rapid movement that caused the muscle spasm. This position will relax the spastic, painful muscle by shortening it. Sometimes you might find it necessary to exaggerate that position. This is especially true if the exaggerated position feels more comfortable and the pain in the tender spot continues to improve.

To find this position, you can lie down, Figure 3; sit, Figure 4; or stand, Figure 5. If standing, you might need to rest your arm on a table for support.

Bring your right knee up toward your chest. Move (adduct) the foot, knee, and thigh slightly toward the center of the body. Bend sideways at the waist, slightly to the right. Fine tune this position to find the "sweet spot."

Fold and Hold for at least ninety seconds. Then release slowly.

You can also find this position by kneeling, which

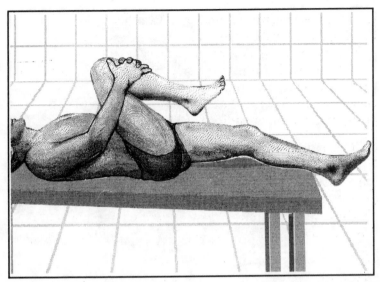

Figure 3 *Fold and Hold* for (iliopsoas muscle)low back pain—lying position.

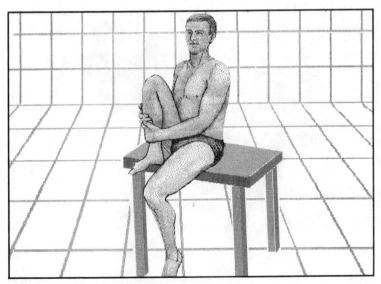

Figure 4 *Fold and Hold* for (iliopsoas m.) low back pain—sitting position.

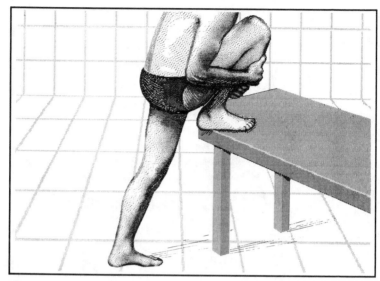

Figure 5   *Fold and Hold* for (iliopsoas m.) low back pain—standing position.

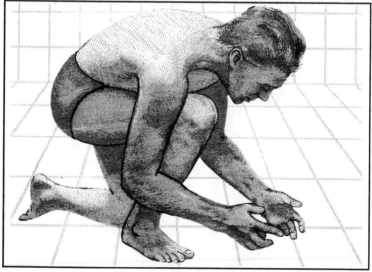

Figure 6   *Fold and Hold* for (iliopsoas muscle) low back pain—kneeling position.

would be very similar to the position you'd assume while gardening, Figure 6.

    Fold and Hold for at least ninety seconds. Then release slowly.

Back pain: Low back/abdomen pain that feels better with sitting

Possible causes

I believe low back pain is so common because many of us sit in a slouched position when lounging or resting. For example, athletes sitting on the bench are often in the "jock position"—bent forward with the forearms resting on the thighs.

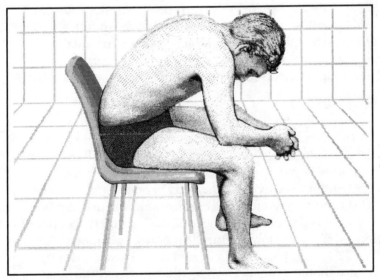

Figure 7 Sitting in the "jock" position.

    In this position the small muscles to the front of the spinal vertebrae and the abdominal muscles are shortened and relaxed. Then, if we make a sudden move to stand or jump up, these muscles go into spasm. Often a nagging backache ensues. Spasm in an abdominal muscle is often felt as a back pain, because a major portion of the abdominal muscles is anchored to thick, fibrous tissue in the posterior back.

Symptoms
People with this kind of pain often feel better when they "tuck in" or "ball up"—that is, when they bend forward at the waist. These people commonly report that standing, walking, or arching their backs makes the pain worse. This happens because such activities passively stretch the spastic muscles.

Find the tender spot
Often people will say that the whole lower back or abdomen aches, and they are not aware of specific tender spots. In addition, it is often impossible to touch the muscles on the front of the spine because the stomach is a formidable barrier (more so in some people than in others). So, the tender spots involved in this pain may be impossible to find.

Fold and Hold
Again, the key to finding a comfortable position is following Mother Nature's clues. If sitting feels better than standing, then do "one better" and tuck. Curl up into a ball by bringing your knees up to your ears or chest and hugging your legs. Try bending and twisting the body to one side or the other to "fine tune" for comfort. If a comfortable position can be found, it is the fold. Hold the position for ninety seconds or longer and very slowly return to a normal position.

You may have to experiment here. Place one leg up higher than the other. Twist a little one way or the other. Bend a little one way or the other. Pay attention to what feels good. Let the "spirit move you." Listen as your body speaks.

For this kind of low back pain, I often instruct the person to find the most comfortable position and rest for up to ten minutes—no matter how grotesque. If you feel silly— who cares? Do you feel better? That's what counts!

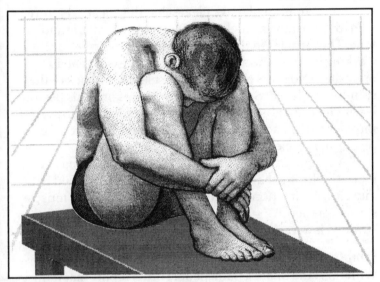

Figure 8   *Fold and Hold* for low back/abdomen pain that feels better with sitting.

Back pain: Low back/abdomen pain that feels better with standing

Possible causes
Often people complain of low back pain that feels better when they stand or walk. They can usually feel a tender spot in the muscles on the posterior, or back side, of the vertebrae (back of the back). There are many of these muscles. Some are very short, functioning only between neighboring vertebrae. Others bridge two or three vertebrae, and still others extend the whole length of the back.

These muscles arch the back and keep the spine in an upright position. When functioning normally, they are strong enough to keep us from slouching. These muscles go into spasm when they are suddenly lengthened from the reflexly relaxed position.

An example will make clear what this means. Picture someone pushing a stuck car out of a snow drift or mud hole. The muscles to the front of this person's spine are working hard. At the same time, those muscles that do the opposite action (the antagonist muscles to the back of the spine) are relaxed. Suddenly the car moves and this person lunges forward abruptly, rapidly lengthening the posterior muscles to the back of the spine. This rapid lengthening results in muscle spasm.

A second cause of this type of back problem may be repetitive lifting that strains these poorly conditioned back muscles. As mentioned earlier, one of the causes of muscle spasm is repetitive strain—especially if the muscle being strained is a weak one.

Symptoms
With this kind of back pain, people often report that it hurts to sit or bend forward. This action stretches the muscles that are in spasm. Bending forward to pick up an object from the floor hurts because the muscles are stretched. Lifting the object and straightening up elicits more pain because these muscles are then required to work. Working over a work bench or counter, making beds, or vacuuming often feel uncomfortable. Common daily activities both work and stretch these spastic muscles, provoking pain.

Find the tender spot
You can usually find tender spots in the back near the spine. One or more muscles may be in spasm, so several tender spots can be present on one or both sides of the back.

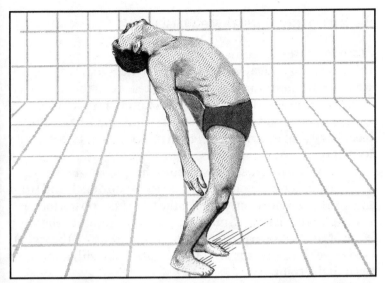

Figure 9   *Fold and Hold* for low back/abdomen pain that feels better with standing.

Fold and Hold

If you have this kind of back pain, you'll often find that it feels better to stand, sit up straight, or walk. Women will usually feel better in high-heeled shoes; walking or arching the back helps relieve their pain. All these comments are clues to finding a comfortable position for *Fold and Hold*.

Standing with your back to a table or other piece of furniture, fold by arching the back backward. Twist and bend toward (or 10 percent away from) the tender spot until the pain diminishes and the position feels comfortable. Lying on your stomach while propped up on your elbows or hands may also be a comfortable position. *Fold and Hold* for at least ninety seconds. Then release slowly.

Back pain: Rotating-at-the-waist pain

Possible causes

Back pain may not always originate in the middle of the back. A common complaint is flank ache, pain that worsens when you bend or twist to the side. This is a problem for many athletes, and I see it mostly in tennis, baseball, and basketball players. However, such pain can also come from "out of the blue."

I believe the muscle involved is the quadratus lumborum. It runs from the lowest ribs in the back and from several of the lower vertebrae to the top of the posterior part of the pelvic crest. This muscle is part of the crest of the wing bone of the pelvis. The function of this muscle (on the right) is to bend the body sideways to the right, and with a slight twist to the right.

This muscle can go into spasm when you:

- Sit or sleep in a position where you're bent or twisted to the right and suddenly straighten or move to your left. When you do this, you suddenly lengthen muscles that were in a shortened, relaxed position.

  As another example, the "batter's box" stance of the baseball player places the quadratus lumborum in a relaxed state. This muscle may go into spasm when the batter "swings for the fence" and goes all the way around, or "wiffs." The player may experience a sudden painful muscle "strike."

- Push a heavy object forward and to the left while you are twisted and bent to the left. Suddenly the object you're pushing moves and you lunge to the left. The right quadratus lumborum muscle, which is reflexly relaxed, is suddenly lengthened and reacts by going into spasm.

- Repeatedly load the quadratus lumborum muscle by rotating and bending to the right. This irritates the muscle and may result in a spasm. An example of such motion is old-fashioned "fire bucket brigade" movement, which requires you to pass the water bucket from left to right.

Symptoms
The pain in stretching the spastic muscle occurs when you bend and twist to the left. Loading and working the muscle will cause pain if you try to push a heavy object toward the right side with your shoulder or do the fire bucket brigade with a left-to-right movement. A deep breath may also aggravate the discomfort because of the muscle's rib attachments.

Find the tender spot
The tender spot is in the lower back, below the ribs and to the side, in the flank area.

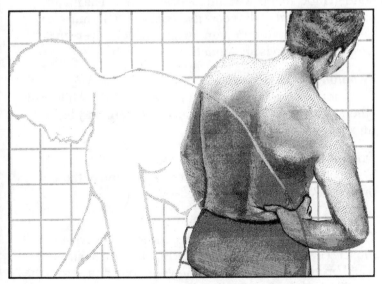

Figure 10 *Fold and Hold* for rotating-at-the-waist pain. (Shadow indicates position of painful lengthening.)

Fold and Hold

Bend and twist your trunk toward the right, finding a position that erases the tender spot. If necessary, do some fine tuning: Experiment with slightly different positions until you find the most comfortable one—the sweet spot. The position you settle on may appear "funny." Don't worry about that. Just maintain this fold. Hold for ninety seconds and very slowly release. Afterwards, gently stretch in the opposite (mirror-image) direction.

Back pain: Tailbone (coccyx pain)

Possible causes

Tailbone pain can be a real "pain in the rear end." Often it is associated with a "prattfall," but it can also come from other sudden movements we tend to forget about. The major cause is a spasm in the coccygeus muscle. This muscle is part of the pelvic diaphragm muscle, which covers the "floor" of the pelvis and attaches to the tailbone (coccyx).

Symptoms

Common reports include "My tailbone hurts" or "It hurts when I sit down." Having a bowel movement may feel uncomfortable.

Find the tender spot

You'll often find tenderness at or near the end of the spine, on one side or the other of the coccyx.

Fold and Hold

The fold that shortens and relaxes the right coccygeus muscle can be done lying or standing. In both positions, you'll bring your right leg behind your body and across the middle of the body toward the opposite side.

To treat a tender spot on the right side of the coccyx, lie on your left side on the edge of a bed. Place your back near the edge of the bed. Flex your left leg upward, resting on the bed for stability. Then bring your right leg behind the body (hyperextended) and allow it to fall toward the floor (adducted). Fine tune this position until the tender spot goes away. You may need to twist your thigh slightly in one direction or the other.

You can assume the same position while standing, which allows for additional adduction of the leg if needed. If the tender spot does not erase in this position, do the same movement but with the left leg behind the body.

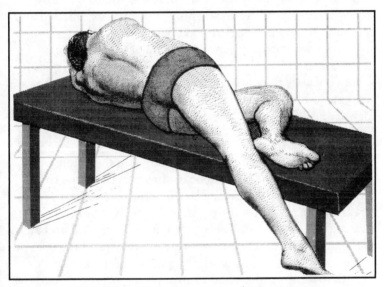

Figure 11   *Fold and Hold* for tailbone pain—lying position.

Remember that in an effective *Fold and Hold*, the tender spot is at least 75 percent lessened. The position, while perhaps awkward, feels comfortable. *Fold and Hold* for at least ninety seconds. Then release slowly.

Back pain: Upper back

Possible causes
One of the most common complaints I hear, especially from people who work at a desk or a counter, involves pain in the upper back. Often the same thing happens with people who spend much of the day being "couch potatoes" (or if very young, "tater tots").

When you sit or stand in a slouched position, your upper back is rolled forward. The muscles on the front of the upper (thoracic) spine are relaxed. If you suddenly move from this position, these "sleeping" muscles are startled and can go into spasm. The slouched position can also lead to stretching and consequent weakening of the muscles posterior to the spine. These weakened muscles can go into spasm because they are constantly being strained by the struggle to hold up the weight of a head that's jutting forward.

Symptoms
Small muscles of both the flexor group and the extensor group of the upper back can be in spasm at the same time. This pain may be aggravated by movement in either direction because of multiple muscle involvement. With this type of pain just the simple attempt to stand up tall and align the "ear and the rear" can provoke pain by stretching spastic flexor muscles—and by working spastic extensor muscles.

Over years, a slouched posture, if uncorrected, leads to the slumping "little old lady" or "little old man" posture with rounding of the whole back, the upper back "hump" and the chin and head jutting forward.

Find the tender spot
There may be multiple tender spots in the upper back and neck. You may need to fold, hold, and then stretch each of them. It's possible, though, that you may not be able to feel all the tender spots.

Fold and Hold

Relief for some upper back pain sometimes comes when you exaggerate the slouched position for ninety seconds and then slowly stand up tall. More frequently, however, you can alleviate the upper back pain and tender spots by arching the back. *Fold and Hold* for at least ninety seconds. Then release slowly.

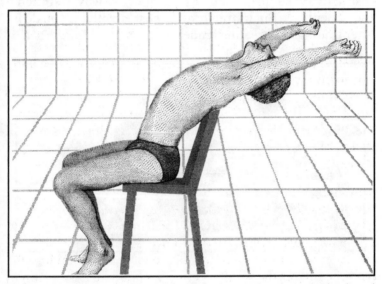

Figure 12   *Fold and Hold* for upper back pain—arching the back and stretching for upper back pain.

For some of the tender spots found in this kind of back pain, you may want to fold away from them instead of over them. Try both ways. Whatever relieves pain and erases the tender spot is correct. You might need to *Fold and Hold* for ninety seconds in several slightly different positions to relax muscles at different vertebral joints.

Relaxing the spastic spine muscles is crucial, but it's

only part of the solution. Stretching the tight, shortened tissues and strengthening the stretched, weakened back muscles is also necessary.

Stretch by arching over the back of a chair. This is another example of following Mother Nature's clues. After a long session of working at a desk, many of us do this stretch spontaneously and think, "Oh, that hurts sooo good." This instinctive wisdom is our clue to an effective way to stretch the upper back. Such stretching is most effective if you do it after finding and treating tender spots with *Fold and Hold*.

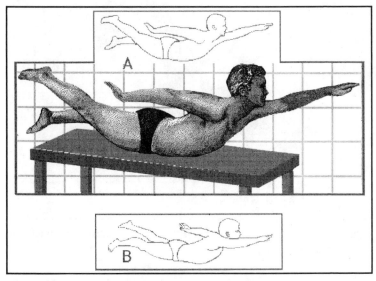

Figure 13   The swimmer's exercise.

After stretching the upper back, do an exercise to strengthen it. I recommend the "swimmer's exercise." Lie face down on the floor. Raise your right arm and left leg, then return them to the floor with the right arm extended above the head and the left arm at the side. Reverse arm position, next, raise your left arm and right leg, then return them to the floor. Alternate these movements and repeat for five minutes. This exercise is effective whether you move slowly or rapidly.

Plan the exercise for when you're doing something else, such as watching television.

Maintaining good posture is the key to keeping youthful flexibility in your upper back. For more ideas on how to do so, see Chapter Five.

Buttocks/back tightness and pain (piriformis muscle spasm with or without sciatica)

Possible causes

Low back pain and sciatica is common in joggers, runners, and power walkers. People can be incapacitated by this condition, which often includes pain and numbness that radiates to the leg. (Sciatica refers to pain down the leg.) Many patients I see have had extensive workups with unnecessary x-rays or CAT scans and MRIs (magnetic resonance imaging) that show no significant abnormality. Often they've tried physical therapy and medications, without success.

After I question them closely, I usually find out these people are not talking about back pain. Instead, they are talking about buttock pain radiating to the back and leg. I usually find a very tender spot in the mid buttock, right in the piriformis muscle.

The piriformis muscle is about the size of a hot dog and originates in the pelvis on the front side of the sacral bone. This muscle attaches to a point on the upper outer region of the femur (large leg bone). You use the piriformis to rotate your leg outward and flex it slightly at the hip.

The sciatic nerve lies deep under the piriformis as the nerve passes over a bony ridge of the pelvis. When the piriformis muscle is in spasm, it squeezes against this bony ridge and pinches the sciatic nerve against this hard surface. The resulting injury and bruising of the nerve results in leg pain, numbness, or both.

A person with piriformis muscle spasm often walks bent forward slightly to the right. The knee and hip are slightly flexed, and the leg and foot are rotated slightly outward.

The piriformis muscle is relaxed when you sit or sleep with a leg in the "frog position." This is the position you assume when you sleep on your stomach and bring your knee up and out to the side. Many people also assume this position when driving long distances in a car with the cruise control on. Here the right leg is spread out to the side, and the foot may be resting up on the center floor divide.

Moving quickly from the "frog position" during sleep or upon awakening can result in piriformis spasm. The same thing can happen if you need to brake suddenly while driving with the leg resting in this position.

Symptoms
Tender spots in the right buttock can feel painful in a sitting position. For this reason, the person in pain tends to put more weight on the left buttocks when sitting. Working the piriformis muscle by pushing the knee outward while you're in the sitting position will also cause pain in the buttocks.

Stretching the spastic piriformis seems to aggravate the symptoms. Walking up stairs feels worse than walking down them. Crossing the right leg over the left is painful. Prolonged standing or walking makes pain worse.

Find the tender spot
You can usually find a tender spot of the piriformis muscle in the middle of the buttock. (For anatomists, this is halfway between the posterior superior iliac spine of the pelvis and the greater trochanter of the femur.)

Fold and Hold
You can usually alleviate buttock pain by putting your foot up on a stool while standing. Draping the leg over the arm of

a chair will also give some relief. So will sitting with your foot up on a chair or couch and letting the leg and knee fall outward. Often the person in pain will say that sleeping with the leg out to the side in the "frog position" feels comfortable.

Fold and Hold in this condition means assuming the "frog position" and fine tuning it so that the tender spot goes away. You can do this while lying on your stomach, lying on your back, or standing. For the stomach position, you may need to ask someone to help you *Fold and Hold*.

In each case, *Fold and Hold* for at least ninety seconds. Then release slowly.

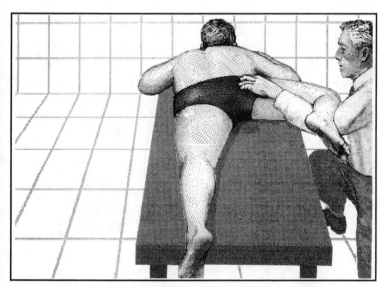

Figure 14   *Fold and Hold* for buttocks /back pain—lying on stomach.

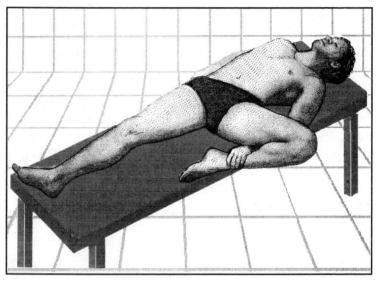

Figure 15 *Fold and Hold* for buttocks/back pain—lying on back.

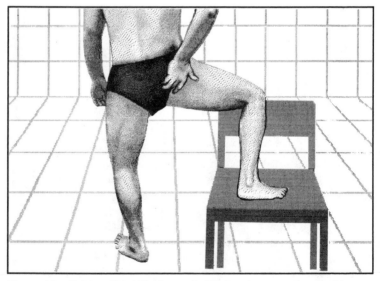

Figure 16 *Fold and Hold* for buttocks/back pain—standing position.

Be sure to follow this *Fold and Hold* treatment with stretching of the piriformis muscle. Do this by getting on your hands and knees in the "cat position." For a right-sided buttock pain, bring your left leg over the right leg and move your left buttock toward the right foot. You will feel a tight pull in the right buttock as the piriformis stretches. Repeat three times.

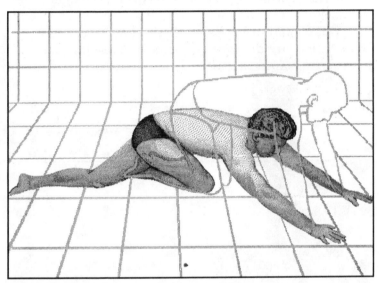

Figure 17   Stretching piriformis muscle after the *Fold and Hold* for buttocks/back pain.

Elbow pain: Golfer's elbow

Possible causes

"Golfer's elbow" is frequently due to a spasm in one or more of the flexor muscles in the forearm and wrist. These muscles are on the front of the forearm and attach to the bony prominence at the inner elbow. The technical name for this prominence is the medial epicondyle of the humerus.

The flexor muscles of the forearm can go into spasm when lengthened suddenly from a relaxed position, where the wrist and elbow were markedly flexed. This is a common sleeping position. Repetitive lifting that flexes the elbow, forearm, and wrist can also lead to spasm of these forearm flexor muscles. Examples of this movement include directing traffic to "come through," as well as sorting and lifting small objects and throwing them over the right shoulder.

This condition is called "golfer's elbow" because new golfers often hit a divot instead of the ball, resulting in sudden strain and spasm of this muscle group.

Symptoms
Symptoms of golfer's elbow include tenderness and pain over the inside of the elbow. Pain is worse when the flexor

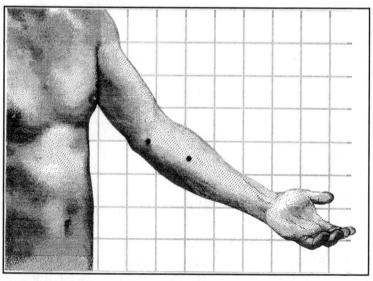

Figure 18   Tender spots for golfer's elbow.

muscles are loaded or worked as described above. Passively, extending the elbow, wrist, and fingers stretches these muscles and causes added pain if they are in spasm.

Find the tender spot
Tender spots for golfer's elbow are usually on the inside of the elbow (toward the body). Sometimes you can also find tender spots in the front of the forearm or wrist.

Fold and Hold
Treatment for golfer's elbow is the same as that for the wrist pain known as carpal tunnel syndrome (page 94). The *Fold and Hold* position for this pain is similar to the position you used as a child to make "swan shadows" on the wall. At first it seems complicated, but once you do it a couple of times, it becomes easy.

Bend your arm up and touch your shoulder with your fingertips. Now turn your hand and fingers outward 180

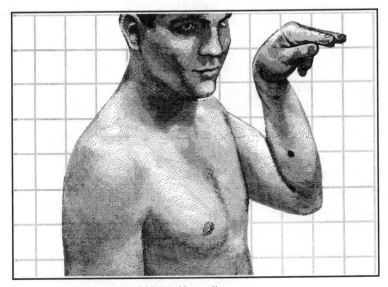

Figure 19 *Fold and Hold* for golfer's elbow.

degrees from your shoulder in a clockwise direction. Flex your wrist and cup your hand downward slightly. Point your thumb and fingertips toward the floor. You might need to use a slight force outward and/or downward on the hand.

Find the position where your tender spot goes away. If needed, fine tune this position by moving your hand a little to the left, right, up, or down. Hold this position for ninety seconds. It is quite common for the hand to fall asleep in this position. Unless it is painful, this is no cause for concern. Just keep holding the fold. *Fold and Hold* for at least ninety seconds. Then release very slowly.

Elbow pain: Tennis elbow

There are several forms of so-called tennis elbow. The following treatment is for one of the most common forms.

Possible causes

Tenderness over the outer prominence of the elbow is called "tennis elbow"—in all likelihood because it bothers many who pursue this sport. But this is a problem that results from many other pursuits as well.

Tennis elbow is often caused by spasm and tightness of the extensor muscles of the forearm, wrist, and hand. A spasm in an upper forearm muscle that twists the forearm outward (the supinator muscle) frequently contributes to the pain. All these muscles attach to the outer, bony prominence of the elbow. In medical terminology, this prominence is called the lateral epicondyl of the humerus, and the tenderness of tennis elbow is called lateral epicondylitis.

Symptoms

Pain and tenderness can be found on the outer backside or outer front of the elbow region. Less frequently, you can find it in the muscles or tendons on the back of the arm, wrist, or hand. This pain is often aggravated when you work the extensor or supinator muscles with straightening and outward twisting activities of the arm. This means that pain can occur while turning doorknobs, turning screwdrivers, wringing cloths, or washing walls. Pain comes from a clockwise working movement in a right-sided problem. Such movements, for the most part, give pain because they actively load the spastic muscles. This loading also occurs when lifting objects with the elbow bent and the palm toward the floor or when holding up the wrist and forearm while writing with a pen or typing.

Pain can also be elicited or aggravated by passive stretching of the extensor muscles by flexion of the wrist, forearm, and elbow as in the "swan position." (This position is the fold treatment for "golfer's elbow"; see Figure 19.) These muscles are also passively stretched with such activities as a tightening of the hand grip while shaking hands or lifting a heavy coffee mug to the mouth. People

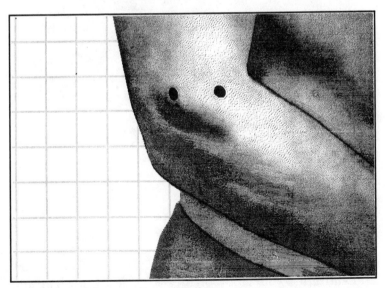

Figure 20   Tender spots for tennis elbow.

with tennis elbow find that their grasp is weak and unreliable (particularly when grasping large objects) and items fall from their hands.

Find the tender spot

You can usually find a tender spot over the outer back side or outer front of the elbow. Feel along the back side of the elbow first. If you don't find it there, then keep moving toward the front. You may find tender spots on the back of the forearm or wrist as well.

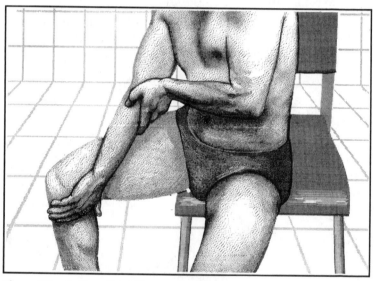

Figure 21   *Fold and Hold* for tennis elbow.

Fold and Hold

Do this sitting in a chair. Twist your right arm outward in a clockwise direction. Your thumb should be facing downward and your palm will be outward. Place your thumb and palm on the inside of your right knee. Using your left hand, grasp your elbow on the back side and push up and outward to the right, overextending the elbow.

You might feel a somewhat uncomfortable stretch sensation in the front of the arm. Endure this for ninety seconds, as long as the discomfort is not over a 3 on a scale of 0 to 10. Then release slowly.

Foot pain: Bunion pain

Possible causes

This problem is common among women who wear pointed, tight, high heels. The shoe pushes the big toe toward the center of the foot and tends to roll the toe under the foot. The adductor hallucis brevis, a foot muscle, is maximally shortened and relaxed ("asleep") when the shoe forcefully squeezes the forefoot and the toes into this unnatural position. By the end of the day, the rest of the now swollen, pinched foot is in pain. This gives rise to the often-heard complaints "My feet are killing me" and "I can't wait to kick off these shoes."

Kicking off the shoes allows sudden lengthening and "awakening" of the adductor hallucis brevis. The muscle responds by going into spasm. When this muscle is activated or in spasm, it pulls the big toe into the position associated with a bunion.

Symptoms

The pain over the bony prominence—the bunion—is due to a bursitis or inflammation that results from the rubbing of the tight shoes. People with bunions commonly experience even more pain in the ball of the foot—particularly when walking barefoot or in sandals.

Find the tender spot

The tender spot to be monitored during *Fold and Hold* treatment is not over the bony bunion prominence. Instead, it is on the ball and bottom of the big toe. This is where the muscle in spasm attaches.

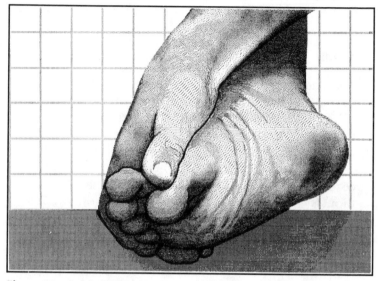

Figure 22   *Fold and Hold* for bunion pain.

Fold and Hold

To treat this pain, exaggerate the bunion deformity. Twist the big toe under the foot and push outward toward the center of the foot. Do this by yourself, or with help from another person. It looks painful, but it often feels goooood. *Fold and Hold* for at least ninety seconds. Then release slowly.

Foot pain: Heel pain/spur (spasm of the flexor digitorum brevis)

Possible causes

This variety of heel pain is often referred to as plantar fasciitis by physicians. It is one of the most frustrating and troublesome foot pains we encounter. For many it is a chronic condition, often lasting two to three years, that developed from no apparent injury. Often it is treated with medications, orthotics, heel cups, cortisone injections, and more—with less-than-satisfactory results.

With this heel problem, people feel tenderness and pain at the site where the flexor digitorum brevis muscle attaches on the bottom of the foot at the front base of the heel. This muscles flexes the forefoot and toes toward the floor.

I think there are three causes of this muscle spasm. They are:

- Sleeping on your stomach with the toes pointing down like a ballet dancer, or on your back with heavy bedding pushing down on the tops of your feet. Both positions point the toes downward. Here the flexor digitorum brevis is shortened and relaxed. A sudden, upward movement of the foot may excite it into spasm.

- Pushing up or lifting a heavy object with the forefoot can cause a reflex relaxation of the muscles on the bottom of your foot. Then, a sudden upward movement of the foot could cause a spasm of the sole muscles. This can happen, for example, when you lift a heavy or stuck garage door with your forefoot and toes. If the door suddenly releases, you can send the muscle(s) on the bottom of the foot into spasm.

- Repetitive use of the flexor digitorum brevis muscle may cause spasm. This often happens when people wear loose, flat sandals. They must repeatedly flex the foot and toes during walking to hold the sandals on.

Symptoms
This pain usually feels worse when you wake in the morning and when you start to walk after being off your feet. You can sometimes "walk off" the tenderness for a short time, but it

usually returns and worsens with prolonged walking or standing.

An x-ray of the foot (which is almost always unnecessary) can show a heel spur. The heel spur, however, is not the cause of the heel pain. Instead, the spur results from the pull of the spastic muscle at its site of attachment to the heel bone. It's often difficult, however, to convince someone who sees the visual evidence of a spur on an x-ray that a muscle they can't see is in fact the culprit.

Pain is produced by putting pressure directly on the tender spot. Prolonged standing or walking, however, may result in a type of accupressure that fatigues the spastic muscle and gives some temporary relief. Working or loading the muscle by pushing the toes down against a barrier (walking up stairs) may give some pain. Stretching the muscle by flexing the foot upward may also cause pain.

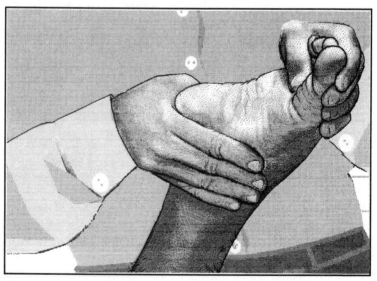

Figure 23 *Fold and Hold* for heel pain/spur —assisted position.

Find the tender spot

The muscle in spasm originates from the bottom front of the heel bone. This muscle inserts at the outer four toes and flexes these toes. It also pulls the bottom of the forefoot toward the heel. I stress again: The spur results from the pull of the tight muscle at its attachment to the heel bone. This is usually where you will find the tender spot. After the muscle is relaxed, the tender spot ceases to be a problem. Eventually even the spur often disappears.

Fold and Hold

To treat this heel pain/spur, fold the bottom of your foot by pushing the heel and toes together. You can get someone to help you with this. Lie on your stomach and bend your knee with the foot toward the ceiling. Ask the other person to push your heel toward the toes and push your toes toward the heel.

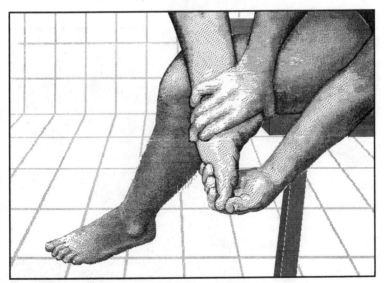

Figure 24 *Fold and Hold* for heel pain/spur—self-treatment in sitting position.

You can also do this treatment by yourself. In a sitting position, bring your right foot to your lap. Push your right heel toward your toes with your right hand. With your left hand, pull the forefoot and toes toward the heel. If you're doing this correctly, you'll see folds in the bottom of the foot. Note: Here you don't have enough hands to touch the tender spot and monitor its relaxation!

From a standing position, you can put the top of the foot on a padded chair and push the heel toward the toes. The chair helps to push the toes to the heel. *Fold and Hold* for at least ninety seconds. Then release slowly.

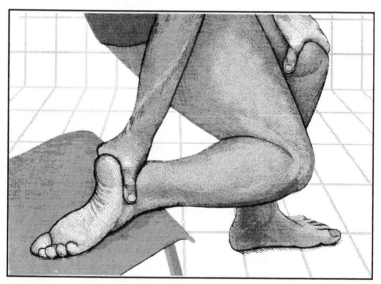

Figure 25   *Fold and Hold* for heel pain/spur—self-treatment in standing position.

After the *Fold and Hold*, stretch the bottom of the foot and calf muscles by standing with the right foot and heel flat on the floor. Place the left foot forward with the knee bent. Lean the body forward, pulling the calf muscle and flexing the foot upward at the ankle. Hold this stretch three or four times for thirty seconds or more. Do it gently, slowly, and without bouncing.

For this condition I also recommend a soft, over-the-counter arch support and an anti-inflammatory medication (such as aspirin, ibuprofen, or a prescription anti-inflammatory) for ten to fourteen days.

Performing this stretch at bedtime will often prevent cramping in the calf, a common complaint of older patients. (I call them "vintage people," or VPs.) Do not confuse these cramps with the muscle spasms you can treat with *Fold and Hold.*

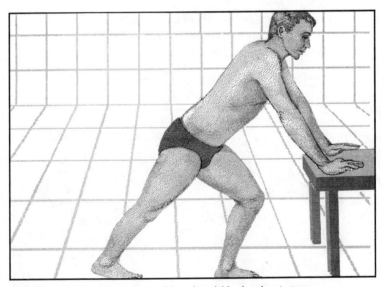

Figure 26 Stretching after *Fold and Hold* for heel pain/spur.

Foot pain: Tenderness on the forefoot (metatarsalgia)

Possible causes
Metatarsalgia results from a spasm in one or several small muscles (the lumbricals and interossei) on the bottom of the foot. These muscles assist in flexing or extending the toes. Metatarsalgia is caused in much the same ways as heel spur pain (see page 66 for more details).

Symptoms
Metatarsalgia is weight-bearing pain (and a subsequent non–weight bearing ache) in the mid-ball of the foot.

Find the tender spot
Look for tender spots on the ball of the foot, or where the muscle attaches to bone. (For you anatomists, this is near the prominent metatarsal head.)

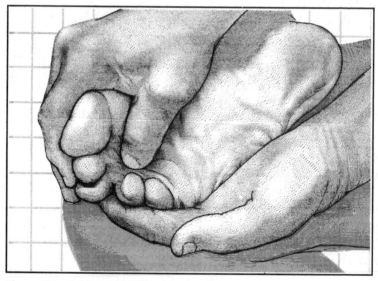

Figure 27   *Fold and Hold* for metatarsalgia.

Fold and Hold
Fold the toes and forefoot toward the tender spot while pulling to "widen" the foot. *Fold and Hold* for at least ninety seconds. Then release slowly.

Hand pain: Weeder's thumb/Tea sipper's thumb

Possible causes
Episodes of hand, finger, or thumb pain represent a common problem. When the pain is not due to an arthritic condition, it is often due to spasms in the small muscles of the hand and wrist.

One example of hand pain is spasm in the adductor pollicis or opponens pollicis muscle. These muscles are located in the "meaty" area at the base of the thumb and the web space. The action of these muscles is to bring the thumb across the palm and allow the pads of the thumb and the fingers to touch—that is, to pinch. These muscles can go into spasm from:

- Rapid movement from a shortened position. This most likely occurs when the thumb is tucked across the palm and the hand is held in a loose fist—a position that often happens during sleep. Sudden opening of the hand can result in a spasm of the startled, sleepy muscles.
- Repetitive, active working of the muscle that comes with pinching-like actions.

Symptoms
When these muscles are in spasm, any use of the pinch grip will elicit pain. It will hurt to hold a pen, button clothing, weed the garden, hold a paint brush, shake hands, or perform similar movements. Pain could also be aggravated by passively stretching the muscles—spreading the thumb away from the hand.

Find the tender spot

You can usually find a tender spot in the "meaty" swelling at
the base of the thumb or in the "web" between the thumb
and forefinger.

Fold and Hold

Fold your thumb over the tender spot. This moves the
thumb into the palm, with the tip of the thumb coming to
the base of the little finger. To maximally relieve the tender
spot, you may need to use your other hand in fine tuning this
position.

An alternate treatment is to place the thumb as
illustrated above and then bring the fingers down into a fist.
Hold the thumb in this folded position for ninety seconds
and slowly release.

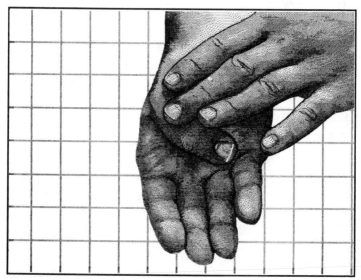

Figure 28   *Fold and Hold* for weeder's thumb hand pain.

Head and neck pain

"Help! I've got a killer headache (neck ache)." This is one of the most frequent complaints heard by a physician. Almost everyone has a headache or neck ache at one time or another. There are several types of headaches, and many factors contribute to them: diet, weather, anxiety, and more. The vast majority of headaches, however, are due to or significantly affected by tight, spastic neck muscles.

Possible causes

As in most muscular pain, the muscles in your neck may go into spasm when suddenly lengthened from a shortened, relaxed, "sleepy" position—or when a weakened muscle has been strained by constant overuse.

Neck muscles may also go into spasm when you straighten your neck rapidly after waking up from an awkward sleeping position. This suddenly "startles" the muscles from a relaxed state. Here's an example: You fall asleep sitting in a chair, with your head falling forward toward your chest. The phone rings. You jerk your head to an upright position and rush to answer the phone. Or, you fall asleep while lying down and watching television. Your head is propped up on a hard pillow or the arm of a couch. Again, your chin is resting on your chest, and your neck is bent and twisted to one side. Someone rings the doorbell, and you leap to attention.

These are just two examples. The rapid return to a normal position from awkward, relaxed positions can occur in many common situations: when responding to an alarm, a baby's cry, a nightmare, or the like. Any of these movements can send shortened, relaxed muscles into spasm.

Weak muscles on the back of the neck also go into spasm easily if confronted with the constant strain of poor posture. Observe people slouching over a desk or counter with the shoulders rolled forward, the upper and lower back rounded, and the head and chin jutting forward. I call this the "little old lady–little old man" position. This posture invites strain and spasm of the posterior neck muscles.

As with back muscles, there are many small and large muscles in the neck. Any of them can go into spasm. It can be almost impossible to isolate and name the exact muscles that are in spasm. Once you find the tender spots, however, you can use *Fold and Hold* effectively.

Symptoms
The head hurts. Neck and shoulders feel stiff. Certain head and neck movements may make the pain worse—for example, moving the head to look downward or to the side. At the same time, some head and neck positions may alleviate the pain, such as bending the head to the side and arching the neck backwards.

A common complaint is that the scalp feels tight, like a taut band. Pain is often worse toward the end of the day and is more frequent after prolonged sitting or bending forward over a workbench. Anxiety aggravates the tight muscles that are already in spasm. And, conversely, anxiety can also tighten these muscles and make them more susceptible to spasm.

Find the tender spot
There may be many tender points in the neck. The key is to find the most painful spots and treat them first. When the most tender spots are gone, the others may just dissipate on their own. (Remember the "mother hen" analogy on page 18.) Better yet, *Fold and Hold* all of the tender spots you can find.

Fold and Hold *for the upper neck: Using the de-tenniser*
I'll discuss treatment of neck pain in two parts: treatment for neck pain at the upper base of the skull, and treatment for the rest of the neck. This is necessary because treatment for the first type of neck pain is a modification of the usual *Fold and Hold* method.

The area of the very top of the neck, at the base of the skull, is difficult to fold. You need to use acupressure to fatigue these muscles before they can be "put to sleep" by the hold. To help fold the muscles in this area, I recommend a simple homemade device that I call a "de-tenniser."

To make this device, you'll need two tennis balls and one nylon stocking leg. Slip the tennis balls into the middle of a common nylon stocking. Tie a tight knot next to each ball so that the two balls are held snug next to each other, and so that a section of the stocking is left on both ends.

Note: Before attempting to use the de-tenniser (or the assisted method that follows), arch your neck backward while sitting and hold this position for one minute. If any dizziness or lightheadedness occurs, then straighten your neck slowly and check with your doctor before attempting to use the de-tenniser. Anyone who is over sixty-five or who has vascular, circulatory, or significant neck arthritis should check with their physician before attempting to use the de-tenniser or to do arching positioning of the neck.

To use your de-tenniser, lie comfortably on your back. Place the de-tenniser behind your neck and lie so that the two balls press on the tender muscles at the junction of the skull and neck. With your hands you may pull gently upward on the two free ends to give more stability and slight pressure at the skull/neck junction.

For more comfort, cushion the de-tenniser in a towel. If you want the head to arch backward more, then place the balls of the de-tenniser up on a riser. A book does nicely.

Rest the full weight of your head on the de-tenniser. Hold this position and relax. As the upper neck muscles fatigue from the weight load of the head, the top of the head will slowly and gently move to the floor; the chin will point more to the ceiling.

When they use the de-tenniser, people often feel an acupressure, "good pain." Sometimes they'll feel a slight worsening of the headache on one side of the head at first.

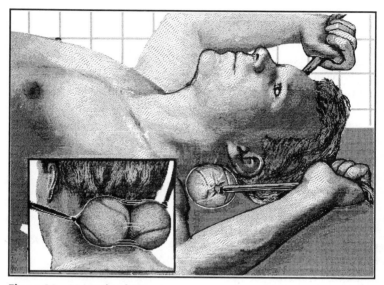

Figure 29   Using the de-tenniser.

Occasionally there may be a minor radiating pain behind the eyes. The "good pain" from the pressure of the balls will slowly improve. Often a sense of general body relaxation follows. Once the pain has been relieved and the neck has folded at this site, hold for at least ninety seconds and then very slowly return to a normal head position.

Headaches caused by tension, anxiety, and poor sitting posture should improve or subside with this method. If the relief is only short-lasting, then look for other tender spots. Consider training yourself to change some habits—specifically, your sitting and standing postures. Look for anxieties that tend to "set up" muscles to spasm. Also concentrate on stretching the tight tissues of the back and strengthening the supportive back and abdominal muscles. For more information on these topics, see Chapter Five.

Assisted Fold and Hold for the upper neck

There are alternatives to using the de-tenniser. The following technique is one of the most wonderfully relaxing things you can do for someone who has a headache or is simply "uptight."

Ask that person to lie comfortably on the floor or bed. Cup your hands so that your finger tips point toward the ceiling and the back of your hands rest on the floor or bed. Have the person in pain lift his or her neck slightly. Slip your cupped hands under the neck. Place your finger tips just below the bony edge of the skull. There are usually tender spots at this site.

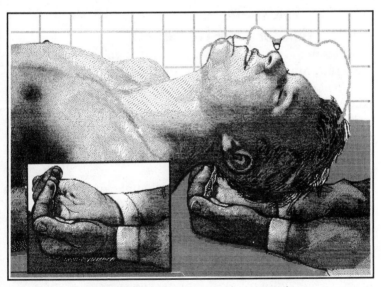

Figure 30 *Fold and Hold* for the upper neck—assisted.

As the other person rests for several minutes with their head/neck junction on your finger tips, that person's tight neck muscles will begin to soften. (Some people say their tense muscles start to melt like butter.) The top of the head will sink backwards, with the chin pointing toward the ceiling.

Here you see the principal of acupressure augmented by *Fold and Hold*. If you merely push on the tender spots—that is acupressure. And acupressure alone will fatigue and relax a spastic muscle to some degree. However, when you additionally shorten the spastic muscles over the fulcrum of the the de-tenniser or the finger tips, you greatly help the muscles relax. Letting the head and neck arch is actually positioning in the fold. After shortening the muscles and encouraging them to rest (hold), one can expect more complete and longer-lasting pain relief than when using acupressure alone.

Fold and Hold for the rest of the neck

Muscles in the mid- and lower neck often go into spasm. Here the pain is referred to as neck and upper back pain.

A common complaint in the emergency department comes from the person who has awakened with a severe pain in the neck. This person presents with the head bent, twisted, and flexed to the side—literally "stuck" in an awkward position. Any attempt to return the head to a normal position is painful.

Again, such muscle spasm can happen when a person awakes suddenly from a nap. Often the person was sleeping with the chin on the right chest and the head bent and twisted to the right. In this position, the muscles in the front and right neck were shortened and relaxed—"sound asleep," so to speak. Then the person suddenly awoke and moved the head rapidly to a normal, upright position. The startled, sleepy muscle awakens abruptly and becomes "irrational." It overreacts to correct the rapid movement. In short, the muscle panics, "hits the brakes," and muscle spasm results.

This violent spasm not only stops the neck from straightening but tends to pull the head back to the sleeping position. Passive movement of the head upward, backward, and to the left will stretch the spastic muscle and cause pain. Working or loading the muscle by having the person push the head down, forward, and to the right against resistance will also increase the pain.

In these cases, you can usually find tender spots on the right side of the neck. Though there may be several, one tender spot is usually much worse.

Treatment in this case is a relaxing, passive fold over the tender spot. Move toward the awkward comfortable sleeping position—the position the head and neck were in prior to the muscle spasm. It may even be more effective to exaggerate that sleeping position—that is, to fold the neck and head even farther forward and toward the right than they were originally. Usually this erases the tender spot and gives comfort.

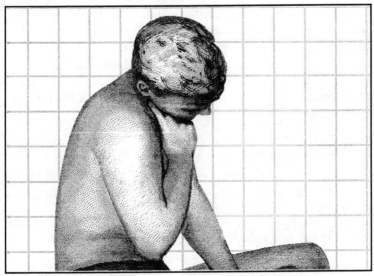

Figure 31 *Fold and Hold* for mid/lower neck pain (one of many possibilities).

This comfortable position may feel awkward and appear unusual. Don't worry—it's still effective.
Fold and Hold for ninety seconds. Then release slowly.

Note: After performing any of the neck *Fold and Hold* treatments, stretch your neck in the opposite direction of the fold. For more details, see the instructions for the relaxing stretch on page 105.

Hip pain (tensor fasciae latae muscle spasm)

Possible causes
Athletes involved in the "kicking sports" (such as football and soccer) and hurdlers in track commonly experience outer hip pain. This pain is worse when they move the thigh and leg out to the side. Often it's diagnosed as, or frequently associated with, trochanteric bursitis of the hip.

Such pain is caused by a spasm of the tensor fasciae latae muscle, which moves (abducts) the thigh and leg outward. When you sleep with the leg abducted (out to the side), this muscle is relaxed. As you know by now, a sudden movement from such a relaxed position can lead to muscle spasm. Repeatedly lifting the leg out to the side can also bring on an overuse muscle spasm. This repetitive lifting is the mechanism for most sport-related spasms of the tensor fasciae latae.

Symptoms
Symptoms of this pain include tightness and tenderness over the right hip and upper outer thigh. It hurts to lie on the affected side because of pressure on the tender spot. Actively lifting the leg out to the side, or pushing the thigh or foot out to the side in an attempt to slide something across the floor, is painful. It also hurts to do the "jumping jack" exercise. Passive lengthening of the spastic muscle aggravates the muscle soreness when you cross the right thigh over the left. On the other hand, it usually feels better to rest the leg out to the side on a raised support.

Find the tender spot

You'll usually find tenderness over the outer hip prominence (for you anatomists, the greater trochanter of the femur). Tender spots in the muscle can occur halfway down the outer aspect of the thigh.

Fold and Hold

To apply *Fold and Hold*, bring the leg out from the side of the body and fold at the hip. Place your foot with the inner ankle on a chair. Fine tune this fold by moving the body up or down, forward or backward, until the tender spot goes away. *Fold and Hold* for at least ninety seconds. Then release slowly.

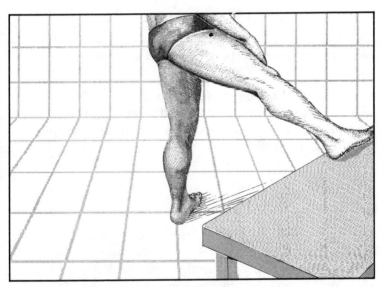

Figure 32   *Fold and Hold* for outer hip pain.

After *Fold and Hold*, lengthen the tensor fascia latae muscle by stretching it in the mirror-image opposite direction from the fold position. To do this, stand several

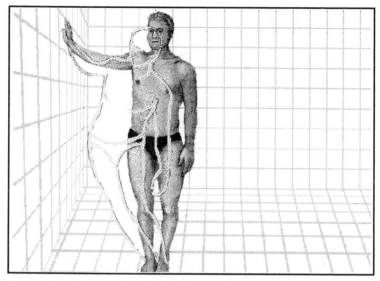

Figure 33 Stretching after *Fold and Hold* for outer hip pain.

feet away from a wall with your right hip toward the wall, brace yourself with your right hand against the wall. Keeping your feet stationary, move your upper body and right hip to the wall.

Shin splints

Possible causes
Running or walking, particularly over long distances in shoes with poor arch support, can cause one type of shin splints. So can getting up rapidly from the "kindergarten style" or "Indian chief" sitting position. This position involves sitting on the floor with the knees and thighs rolled outward and the feet folded inward.

Symptoms
People with the most commonly occurring type of shin splints often feel pain along the inner side of the lower leg

when they walk or run. I judge that most episodes of this type of shin splints occur from a spasm of the tibialis posterior muscle or from a spasm in one of the calf muscles called the soleus and gastrocnemius. These muscles move the ankle and foot toward the ground. Pushing off with the toes during the running or walking stride is most troublesome. Straightening the leg at the knee can make the pain worse by passively stretching the spastic muscles, as can flexing the foot upward.

Find the tender spot
Look for the tender spot right in the area of pain: the mid/lower inner leg, immediately behind the tibia (leg bone). You might find a second tender spot in the fleshy mid-calf.

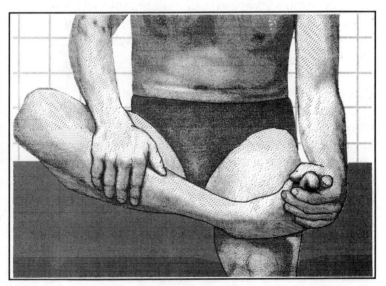

Figure 34 *Fold and Hold* for shin splint—sitting position.

Fold and Hold

You can treat shin splints in a sitting or a standing position. Often sitting is easier.

Sitting position: Bend your right knee and cross your right ankle over the left thigh and rest the ankle on the left thigh. Place your right thumb or finger on the tender spot to monitor it. Extend and invert the right foot, using the left hand to pull the toes toward your face. Fine tune this position until the tender spot is 75 percent improved or gone. *Fold and Hold* for at least ninety seconds. Then release slowly.

Standing position: This position is especially useful if a tender spot is found in the calf (in the gastrocnemius or soleus muscles).

Stand near a table or chair that you can use as a support. Bend your right knee and grab the toes of the right foot with your left hand. Let the heel of the right foot come to rest against the left buttock. Point the toes of your right

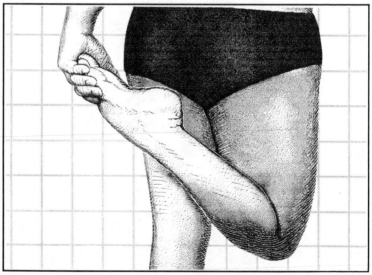

Figure 35   *Fold and Hold* for shin splint—standing position.

foot toward the ceiling. Fine tune in this position until the tender spot is 75 percent improved or gone.

Note: The standing *Fold and Hold* position is also useful for upper posterior heel pain, often diagnosed as Achilles tendonitis. *Fold and Hold* for at least ninety seconds. Then release slowly.

Other notes on shin splints

People with shin splints often benefit from supplemental treatment. Use over-the-counter, soft arch supports in all your shoes. This can reduce the chances of recurring shin splints. In addition, wear soft-heeled and soft-soled shoes. Applying ice prior to an activity can help reduce the inflammation and muscle spasm. Anti-inflammatory medication is often useful.

Shoulder pain: "Pouring the coffee" pain (tendonitis biceps brachii)

Possible causes

This shoulder pain centers on a muscle in the arm and shoulder known as the biceps brachii. Sudden or repeated use of this muscle can send it into spasm.

Symptoms

People with this type of pain feel an ache in the upper front shoulder. Occasionally pain radiates to the back of the shoulder and/or to the front of the arm and elbow. They feel weakness and pain when lifting the arm and hand above the head. Such pain is made worse with activities that involve lifting a weight with the palm forward and up: writing and typing, shoveling snow, serving at tennis, turning a car steering wheel, twisting a doorknob or screwdriver, and the like.

This pain is also made worse with passive stretching of the upper arm. This takes place when you extend your arm backward, rotated slightly outward at the shoulder and moved (adducted) toward the midline of your back. In this position, the elbow is straight and the forearm rotated outward, with the palm facing out and the thumb pointing back.

Find the tender spot
Look for tender spots on the front of the arm an inch above the elbow, in the belly of the biceps. Also look on the bony prominence just beneath the outer end of the collarbone or over the front, outer, upper prominence of the shoulder where the two tendons of this muscle are located.

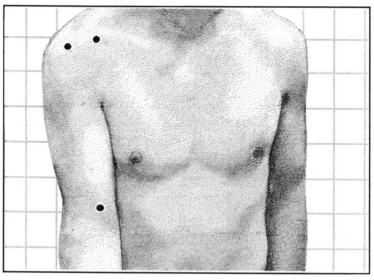

Figure 36   Tender spots for "pouring the coffee" biceps shoulder pain.

Fold and Hold
Fold with the back of the wrist or forearm resting on the forehead. This position flexes the elbow and rotates the upper arm slightly inward at the shoulder. Your palm faces upward (away from your face). Fine tune this position until the tender spot is 75 percent improved or erased. Pushing or pulling inward on the shoulder with the opposite hand to compress the shoulder joint may improve the treatment.

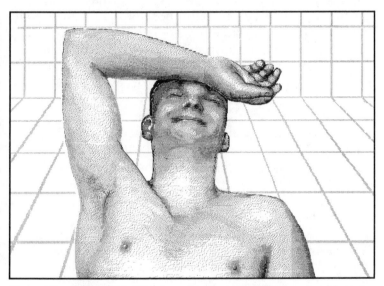

Figure 37   *Fold and Hold* for "pouring the coffee" biceps shoulder pain.

Fold and Hold for at least ninety seconds. Then release slowly.

Shoulder pain: "Putting on a coat" pain

Possible causes
The muscle involved in this variety of shoulder pain is the infraspinatus. It originates from the scapula (wing) bone's

lower, back (posterior) surface. This muscle attaches to the outer, posterior area of the humerus (arm bone), one to two inches below the top of the shoulder. Its action is to move the upper arm backward and inward, and to twist the upper arm outward at the shoulder.

This muscle can go into spasm when you assume the "propped up" relaxed sitting position and then move suddenly. This lounging, sitting position is frequently assumed when sitting on the ground "after a hard game" or at a picnic or at the beach. In this position, you prop up your body by resting it on your elbows or hands with your shoulders rotated outward slightly. Here the infraspinatus is profoundly relaxed. Then a mosquito or a bee lands on your nose, and you make a rapid movement to swat it. This sudden stretch of a relaxed muscle provokes a spasm.

This muscle can also go into spasm when you push up on a heavy object in front of the body—say, a stuck window that is hard to open. As you push up, the infraspinatus muscle is reflexly relaxed. If the window suddenly "lets go" and raises suddenly, this muscle is suddenly lengthened and develops a spasm.

Another possible cause of muscle spasm is repeated backward and twisting actions of the arm at the shoulder. Examples of this movement include paddling a canoe, rowing a boat, cutting grass with a scythe, or spreading grass seed.

Symptoms
With this spasm you'll often feel a deep ache in the front of your shoulder with some pain radiating into the upper arm and neck. You'll find it painful to put on a coat. Women may feel pain when they put on a bra or zip the back of a dress.

The spastic infraspinatus muscle will be passively stretched when you bring your right arm in front of your body and twist it inward to reach or lift something forward and above the left shoulder. Combing your hair or brushing your teeth may be painful. Sleeping on the left side with the right arm resting in front of you on the bed will often cause a painful stretch.

Find the tender spot
Look for a tender spot on the lower part of the wing bone in the back, not near the area where you feel pain in the shoulder. Lying on your back in a position that places pressure on the tender spot will be painful.

Fold and Hold
To find the comfortable fold position, place the arm down at the side and twist it outward, perhaps slightly backward and (adducted) inward toward the center of the body. You may find it helps to have someone else push inward on your shoulder. Or you can pull your shoulder inward with the opposite hand.

You may find yourself sleeping on your right shoulder

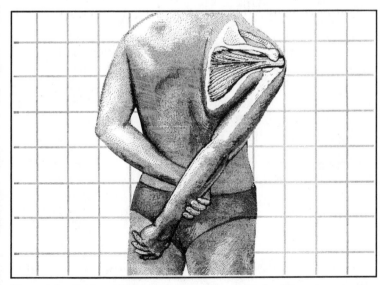

Figure 38 *Fold and Hold* for "putting on a coat" shoulder pain—standing position.

with the right arm behind your back and the palm of your right hand cupping the buttocks. This is Mother Nature's *Fold and Hold* technique. *Fold and Hold* for at least ninety seconds. Then release slowly.

Shoulder pain: "Raising the arm" pain

Possible causes

There are many muscles in the shoulder that may go into spasm and give similar but not quite identical pain. At times several muscles may be involved. Thus, you may need to use several slightly different *Fold and Hold* positions for several different tender spots.

Often pain results from a spasm in the supraspinatus muscle. This muscle goes from the top of the upper scapula (wing bone) to the upper humerus (arm bone). The function of this muscle is to move the arm outward (away from the side of the body) and upward. An example of this movement is raising your hand in class to get the teacher's attention.

This muscle can go into spasm when you fall asleep with your arm raised above your head and then suddenly bring it down to the side. Spasm can also occur when you forcefully push down on an object at your side. Here the muscle can go into spasm when an object you're pushing down on suddenly gives way. Other causes of spasm include repeatedly lifting a light object out to your side, or carrying an object such as a heavy briefcase or suitcase at your side.

Symptoms

When your supraspinatus muscle is in spasm, you may complain of a deep ache in your shoulder that often radiates to the outer elbow. Lifting the affected arm to your side can feel painful. So can raising the arm to brush, curl, or comb your hair. Shaving and brushing the teeth may also cause pain, as can painting, washing walls, cleaning windows, or hanging drapes.

Painful stretching of this muscle occurs when you bring your arm behind your body and upward, toward the center of your back—the "uncle" position. Carrying a weight at the side, even the mere weight of the arm while walking, may aggravate the pain.

Find the tender spot

Tender spots for this muscle may be difficult to find because they are beneath several bony prominences of the shoulder or deep in the thick (upper back) trapezius muscle.

Fold and Hold

To find a comfortable position, raise your arm above your head in the "teacher, I know the answer" hand-raising position. It will be painful if the arm is brought up (adducted) at the side but more comfortable if raised with the arm going forward. Pull the arm slightly forward with

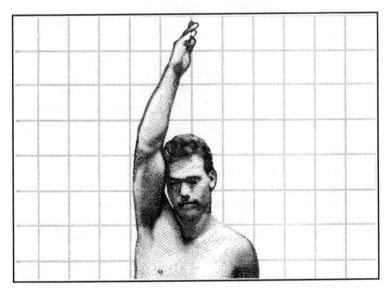

Figure 39   *Fold and Hold* for "raising the arm" shoulder pain.

the thumb toward your back. It often helps to lie on your shoulder or have someone push inward on the shoulder when you're in this "hands-up" position to further shorten the affected muscle. *Fold and Hold* for at least ninety seconds. Then release slowly.

Wrist pain: Carpal tunnel syndrome

Possible causes

Carpal tunnel syndrome is becoming more common today. One reason is that more people work on computers or at jobs requiring repetitive wrist movements. You can also cause this problem by sleeping with your hand and wrist flexed forward (to the palm) and then suddenly moving the wrist straight or into extension when you awake.

In many cases of early carpal tunnel syndrome, *Fold and Hold* has worked effectively. However, in extreme cases, surgery may be needed. As always, I recommend trying *Fold and Hold* first. If after two weeks the pain doesn't go away or it gets worse, see a physician.

Fold and Hold works well as a preventive measure against worsening bouts of wrist pain. If you develop wrist pain, break up your day with ninety-second sessions of *Fold and Hold* relief. Another preventive measure is to stop your work periodically and take breaks. Get up and stretch your wrists in all directions.

Symptoms

With carpal tunnel syndrome, you'll feel pain in the wrist, forearm, hand, and fingers. It is common for the fingers and hand to "fall asleep." The pain is often made worse by extending the hand or wrist, reading a newspaper, driving a car, cupping and twisting the hand outward, receiving coins, using scissors, gripping an object tightly, and the like.

Pulling a cork out of a bottle with your fingers can also be painful.

Find the tender spot

There may actually be more than one tender point in the arm, as more than one of the forearm flexor group of muscles can be in spasm. The most common spots will be along the front (palm side) of the wrist and up the inner front of the forearm. Another possible location could be the inner front of the elbow.

Fold and Hold

The *Fold and Hold* position for this pain is similar to the position you used as a child to make swan shadows on the wall. At first it seems complicated, but once you do it a couple of times, it becomes easy. See treatment for "golfer's elbow," page 61.

Bend your arm up and touch your shoulder with your

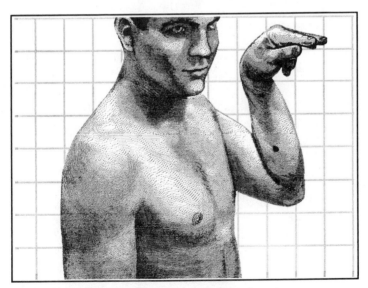

Figure 40 *Fold and Hold* for carpal tunnel wrist pain.

finger tips. Now turn your hand and fingers outward 180 degrees from your shoulder. Cup your hand slightly and point thumb and finger tips toward the floor. Flex your wrist. You may need to use a slight force downward on the back of the hand and you may need to twist inward or outward to fine tune. The tender spot should go away or improve at least 75 percent. Hold this position for ninety seconds. It is quite common for the hand to fall asleep in this position. This is no cause for concern unless the pain worsens. Just keep holding the fold. *Fold and Hold* for at least ninety seconds. Then release slowly.

After treating in the *Fold and Hold* position, stretch the wrist.

4 Common Questions about Fold and Hold

1. When I go to your office, you can position me so I'm comfortable. But how can I do this for myself? Won't it hurt?

No, searching for a more comfortable position can't hurt you. *Fold and Hold* is merely positioning. Again, your reassurance can come from the number of people in discomfort who have fallen asleep and awakened with their pain gone. Mother Nature has put them into a position of comfort—just as you'll do yourself with *Fold and Hold*.

2. I tried* Fold and Hold, *but my pain didn't go away. Why not?

My first question to you would be: Did you find the tender spot? Try again. This time, feel around the pained area until you find the most tender spot. Fold toward and over the spot until the pain subsides and the tender spot significantly lessens or goes away. I call this position the "sweet spot."

Make sure you actually hold this fold for at least ninety seconds. You can hold longer than ninety seconds, but it is very important to hold for at least ninety seconds. Lastly, it is essential that you make sure you release your hold very, very slowly.

You may need to repeat the *Fold and Hold* treatment two or three times a day for three to four days. I tell people that if they are not getting better in this time period (or if they are getting worse), then they should see their physician for another type of treatment.

3. My back hurts, but I can't find a tender spot in my back. Where should I look?

Sometimes the tender spot in back pain is located in the front of the body and not on the back at all. Feel around the lower abdominal muscles and around your pubic bone and groin. Press on the muscles and bony ridges in that area.

Sometimes you are unable to locate the tender spots because they are deep in the abdomen, in the pelvis, or in muscles toward the front of the spine. In this case, forget finding the tender spot. Just concentrate on finding the most comfortable position and holding this position for several minutes. Try to go to sleep in the position of maximum comfort, using pillows to help maintain the position.

4. Can I use Fold and Hold for other pains not in this book?

Yes. *Fold and Hold* should work on any pains associated with muscle spasm. Simply follow the basic techniques: Find the tender spot, fold, and hold for ninety seconds. Return to a normal position slowly.

5. My husband has tennis elbow. Can I do Fold and Hold on him?

Yes, you can often assist another person with this technique. That person may find it easier to get into a comfortable position with your help.

Follow the same basic *Fold and Hold* principles that you use on yourself. Be in constant communication with the person to make sure the pain is getting better, not worse. Remember to monitor the tender spot and to fine tune the position until you find the "sweet spot"—the position where the tender spot is felt only as pressure and the person is comfortable.

6. *What do you mean by "fine tuning"?*
When doing *Fold and Hold*, you use the tender spot as a monitor to help find the most ideal treatment position. Moving the body toward the ideal fold position will lessen tender spot discomfort. When the tender spot becomes pain-free, I call this the "sweet spot."

Remember the safecrackers in old gangster films? They moved the dial on the combination lock slightly to the right or left. Eventually they opened the lock. Like them, you may need to fine tune the fold position—move a little in one direction and then a little in the other until you find the position where the tender spot maximally improves. Even if this position looks awkward, it should be virtually pain-free. (At times you might experience some minor stretch discomfort on the opposite side of the body or limb. This is nothing to worry about.)

7. *What if the tender spot is not located where I feel pain?*
The tender spot is most often where you experience discomfort. But if you've been feeling near the site of pain and you haven't found a tender spot, then look on the opposite side of the body or limb.

This is particularly true with back pains. As an example, the back pain condition that causes you to stand and walk stooped forward and worsens when you try to stand up straight will have no tender spots in the back. Instead, you may find tender spots in your groin, pubic area, or abdominal muscles.

8. *Can* Fold and Hold *be done on senior citizens?*
Yes. Except perhaps for the neck, gently putting someone in a position of more comfort shouldn't be dangerous. Precautions should be used in treating neck pain, particularly the arching positions for people over sixty-five or anyone who

has neck arthritis or head or neck circulation concerns. They should check with a physician prior to using the relaxation device I call the "de-tenniser" or doing other neck treatments (see page 76). In any *Fold and Hold* treatment, no force is used—and if pain is worsened, then STOP.

9. *What are my options when a pain just does not respond to repeated attempts at* **Fold and Hold?**
My estimate is that 75 percent of common aches and pains respond partially or fully to *Fold and Hold*. These are the pains that result primarily from muscle spasm and strained tissue. The remaining 25 percent are often due to old wear-and-tear trauma—infections, tumors, inflammatory conditions, fractures, etc. *Fold and Hold* is not designed for these sources of pain, so see your physician for further treatment.

10. *How often can I do* **Fold and Hold?**
Do *Fold and Hold* three times a day, every day, for two weeks, or until you are no longer in pain. Often you will feel immediate relief. If you are lucky, you may need to *Fold and Hold* only once.

If the pain hasn't significantly improved after one or two attempts, you may need to hunt for other tender spots. If the fold is comfortable, you may find it helps to hold longer than ninety seconds. If you are not feeling better after two weeks, or if at any time you are feeling worse, see your physician.

11. *How soon after doing* **Fold and Hold** *can I start exercising again?*
You can begin exercising almost any time after doing *Fold and Hold*, provided the pain is gone.

I suggest several things to help prevent a return of the spasm. Of greatest importance is gently stretching the treated muscle after the relaxing treatment of *Fold and Hold*. Always stretch in the mirror-image (opposite) position from the relaxing folded treatment position. Using low heat and gentle massage on the involved area after treatment can also help prevent recurring pain. If exercise seems to reactivate the pain, then allow the muscle twenty-four hours of "recovery" rest.

12. *Is* Fold and Hold *the same as acupressure?*
Fold and Hold is an extension of acupressure. The tender spots we look for in *Fold and Hold* are similar to acupressure points. But rather than fatiguing a muscle by applying pressure to the tender spot, *Fold and Hold* puts the muscle into a relaxed position. A spastic muscle that has been rested stays relaxed longer than one that has been simply fatigued.

In a sense, acupressure is "beating" the tender muscle into submission by force, while *Fold and Hold* soothes and coddles the muscle into relaxation.

13. *After relaxing a muscle, is there any special treatment I should give?*
Stretching the muscle that has been relaxed seems to keep pain from recurring. Again, stretch in the mirror-image (opposite) direction from the comfortable position you assumed during *Fold and Hold*. Applying low heat for twenty minutes after each treatment can also help.

14. *Should I be taking aspirin or other anti-inflammatory medication with* Fold and Hold?
Fold and Hold is an approach that emphasizes treating pain without surgery or drugs. However, there are times when it's still appropriate to take over-the-counter anti-inflammatory drugs. If you do, it's important to take these drugs for a full ten days, even if the pain goes away sooner. Otherwise, you end up only putting out the "flames" of the inflammation pain while the "live coals"—the underlying inflammation— still smolder. Just a little wind of provocation may fan the coals and bring the pain back.

Remember to follow directions carefully when taking anti-inflammatory drugs. If your stomach is irritated by these drugs, stop taking them and consult your physician. If you have a sensitive stomach, then taking an enteric-coated (candy-coated) anti-inflammatory pill that dissolves in the small bowel may circumvent this problem. Read all labels carefully.

15. *Is it safe to do* **Fold and Hold** *on children?*

If it's comfortable, it's safe. Mother Nature and kids work cooperatively. Look at the positions that kids assume while sleeping. They do *Fold and Hold* naturally. It's not until we "grow up" that we stop allowing ourselves to be manipulated into awkward positions. Oh, to be a kid again!

While it cannot turn back the clock, *Fold and Hold* can help us regain some of our youthful flexibility. Go for it!

5 Five More Keys to Treating and Preventing Pain

The first step in treating pain resulting from muscle spasm is to use *Fold and Hold*. However, if you want to prevent pain from returning, then understand and apply the five basic specific strategies in this chapter. Use these strategies *in addition* to *Fold and Hold*.

- Do specific exercises to:
  - Stretch the spastic muscle that you treated with *Fold and Hold*.
  - Stretch the tight connective tissue surrounding that muscle.
  - Strengthen weak muscles. (See Diagram 4.)
- Maintain a healthful posture. In fact, if you learn to better manage your sitting and standing postures, you'll learn much about long-term pain relief at the same time.

- Care for your back on a daily basis.
- Allow yourself an optimal amount of pain by learning to distinguish between "good" pain and "bad" pain.
- Work on healing the emotional side of pain.

In this chapter you'll find techniques for accomplishing these goals.

Stretching and strengthening muscles

To gain the full benefit of *Fold and Hold* and to keep from having the same recurring problem, it is imperative to stretch all shortened tissue and strengthen all weak muscles.

Begin by stretching the shortened, previously spastic muscle—the muscle you relaxed by using *Fold and Hold*. Be sure to stretch it in the mirror-image, opposite direction of the fold treatment position.

Any tissue that feels "tight" needs stretching. This should be done gently, slowly, and steadily. When you hold a stretch with full tension and keep a steady pull, you'll often feel a release. This release is the whew! feeling you get when the tissue finally loosens up. This release occurs in the soft connective tissue, both in the muscle and surrounding it.

It's a wonderful sensation when stretched tissues reach a fatigue state and begin to lengthen and "give." It feels like a "melt down." With it often comes a profound sense of relaxation. You can really feel that sensation wash over you as the muscles stop working against the stretching tension. This relaxation at the point of tensile fatigue is what allows you to stretch a bit further each time, and it's a great total body relaxer as well.

Using the relaxing stretch

One of my favorite stretching techniques is also one of the simplest. I call it the relaxing stretch. The relaxing stretch is a comfortable way to gradually increase the length of a muscle and other tight tissue and improve flexibility. This technique will work with any tight muscle or group of muscles. (The instructions below illustrate the stretch using muscles in the right leg and hip.) Here's how to do it:

Step one

Lie on your back and bring the right knee gently toward the chest until it meets slight resistance. This is the first site of tightness, also called the first barrier. There should be minimal or no pain at the barrier.

Step two

After you reach this barrier, do not try to pull the knee any farther toward the chest. Instead of stretching the tight muscles, you are now going to tense and work the muscles.

To do this, place both hands around the knee. Keep your hands stationary and push the knee out against the hands. You're not going anywhere—just tensing the muscles that would normally straighten out the leg.

Note: You are now pushing in the opposite direction of the desired stretch. Make sure that the body stays stationary during this step.

Push the knee outward against your hands for about five seconds.

Step three

Stop pushing and relax.

Step four

Now pull your knee toward your chest. Because you've relaxed muscles that were tense, you can now stretch those muscles a little more. You'll probably be able to move your knee closer to your chest until you reach a new tightness barrier.

Step five
Repeat steps two through four.

The same technique works for any muscle or muscle and joint complex. I have found it especially useful for loosening a tight neck, shoulder, or leg. Each time you push against an unmoving counterforce in the opposite direction from the desired stretch, you work the tight muscle. When you stop pushing, the muscle relaxes. During that brief period of relaxation, you can, with minimal or no discomfort, stretch the muscle to a new barrier.

People who first try this simple technique are usually amazed at how effective it is. Just remember to push against a fixed object in the opposite direction of the desired stretch. Relax, and then move again in the direction you want to stretch—to a new tight barrier. Repeat this whole procedure three or four times. Using the relaxing stretch, you can really become a "loose" man or woman.

Stretching scar tissue
We develop pain for many different reasons. Some of the most common pain is due to scars and stiffness of tight connective tissues. This tight scar tissue needs to be stretched out. Often this means we must go through a period of discomfort to get better.

Scar tissue is like rubber cement poured near the site of an injury. Imagine rubber cement hardening as it dries. Something like this happens to scar tissue that is not stretched.

For another analogy, take a tight piece of rubber or a thick rubber band. If you put this rubber band between your index fingers and start pulling on it, you'll find it takes some work to maintain the stretch. You may even feel slight pain as you pull with your fingers on such tough rubber.

Maintain the pull, however, and that rubber band will eventually soften up.

Scar tissue is like that rubber band. With time it will loosen up, though it may take hard work. To loosen those tight bands of scar tissue that can make movement painful, keep working to stretch. Stay dedicated to your stretching program, even if it means allowing some pain each time you stretch. You may well regain most, if not all, of your ability to move the injured area. Start "pulling for yourself" and your tissue, like the rubber band, can "bounce back."

Another benefit of stretching is that this activity may lengthen and fatigue a tight, spastic muscle. If placed under a constant pull, this muscle may, in time, "give up the fight." In fact, this is the approach initially taken in many pain treatment programs. However, I encourage you to try to use *Fold and Hold* prior to stretching. When you are working with a rested, relaxed muscle rather than fighting an irritated, spastic muscle, the stretch is more effective.

Strengthening muscles

Next, strengthen the weakened, stretched muscle (Muscle B, Diagrams 2 and 3) on the opposite side of the torso or limb from the previously spastic muscle. (See Muscle A, Diagrams 2 and 3.) While both the previously spastic muscle and the opposite, stretched muscle are weak, the lengthened muscle is often weaker. This is particularly true if the pain condition has been long-standing. A weight training program concentrating on the weak muscles should be started. (See Diagram 4.)

Maintaining a healthful sitting posture

When it comes to preventing pain, good sitting posture is crucial. I think poor sitting posture is the key culprit in many of our pains—not just pains in the back and neck but in all areas of the body. Remember the song "Dem bones, dem bones, dem dry bones"? The message is that all parts of our body are connected. A structural dysfunction in one area of the body can result in a dysfunction in another area and consequently a distant pain.

Sitting slouched forward, with a rounded lower back, causes the loss of the inward arch in the low back. That arch is called the lumbar lordotic curve. Loss of this arch by poor sitting posture leads subsequently to the hunched upper back and the neck and chin that jut forward—what I call the "little old lady" or "little old man" back and neck. And this poor sitting and sleeping posture is often responsible not only for low back pain, but for upper back pain, neck aches, headaches, and pain in others of "dem bones" and joints.

Poor posture puts excessive stress on the supporting tissues and bones of the spine. Look at what happens if you sit at a desk all day long. Your head, which weighs about fifteen pounds, places minimal pull or stress on the neck and back muscles when it is high "atop" the spine and you sit tall. In contrast, the slouched posture allows the head to fall forward and the chin to jut forward. Then the pull on the upper posterior neck and back muscles is in effect much more than fifteen pounds. This forward pull causes great strain repercussions on the entire body.

Such strain is unnecessary. By correcting your low back posture you can regain the lordotic curve. The next time you catch yourself sitting and slouching forward, just arch your lower back. See how your neck comes back into a normal, youthful-appearing, statuesque position. The mechanical tension and tugging of muscles in the upper back and neck will be significantly reduced. Your head will once again be realigned with the low back, lessening the pain and tension in the upper back and neck.

When describing this position, I tell people to keep the "rear and the ear" aligned perpendicularly, as in the following illustration.

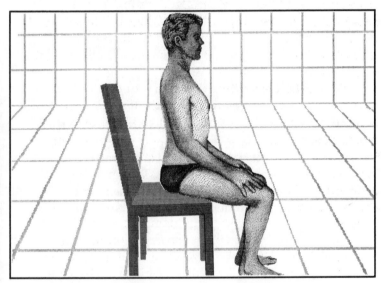

Figure 41   The rear and the ear.

For most people, proper sitting posture is more difficult to maintain than proper standing posture. If we allow poor sitting posture to continue, however, it can affect our standing posture. Therefore it's best to correct sitting posture as early as we can.

Retraining your sitting posture isn't that hard. Work at it diligently for five to six weeks, reminding yourself to arch your lower back whenever you sit. Eventually, your internal computer will "run the program" automatically and will simply make sure you are sitting or standing in a healthful posture. You won't have to remind yourself any longer to sit or stand with an arch in your low back.

The difference this habit makes is amazing. And you can do posture retraining at any age. I've seen eighty-year-old VPs (vintage people) improve their posture significantly.

Poor posture is perpetuated by tight, inelastic tissue. Often this tissue must be loosened before good posture can be attained and maintained. Back-arching exercises (see page 122) can help you work effectively with this tightness.

Using a lumbar roll

To keep that inward arch in your lower back as you sit, use a reminder. One reminder I use is called the "lumbar roll." You can purchase this device in stores, or you can make it yourself. Simply roll up a bath towel and wrap tape around the towel to help maintain the shape. Then put this roll behind your lower back when you sit. Some patients lovingly refer to this homemade device as their "couch potato."

Another option is to make a lumbar roll that can be tied around your waist. Here's how:

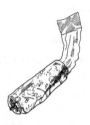

- Take a pair of women's nylon stockings and slide a rolled-up towel into the foot of one of the stockings. (I'll refer to this stocking as stocking 1.)

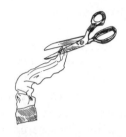

- Then take the other stocking (call it stocking 2) and cut a tiny hole in the toe of it.

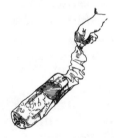

- Next, take stocking 1 and slide the leg end inside the leg of stocking 2. Pull the leg of stocking 1 out through the toe hole of stocking 2.

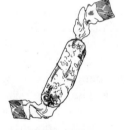

- Now pull stocking 2 all the way through stocking 1 until the rolled-up towel ends up being in the foot of both stockings.

- Finally, tie the leg ends of both stockings around your waist and knot them in the front.

Now you can wear this contraption around your waist. The rolled-up towel will rest in the small of the back, serving both as a support and a reminder to sit up tall. You can even wear it over or under shirts and sweaters. Think of it as a healthful way to "tie one on."

Men who hesitate to wear nylon stockings to the office can ask a physician for a length of stockinette that is used as the first layer of casts. Place a rolled towel in the middle of the stockinette and tie the loose ends of the stockinette around your waist. This way the supportive towel can rest in the lumbar area of your back.

After using some type of lumbar roll as often as possible for a month or so, you'll probably find yourself sitting in a healthful posture automatically.

Exercises to improve posture

In addition to the back-arching exercise explained on page 122, I recommend two other quick exercises for strengthening the stomach muscles. It is difficult to have good posture with weak stomach muscles. Do these exercises when you are on the phone, standing in line, or whenever you think of it. The movements are invisible to other people. No one will ever suspect!

- The "ab in" exercise—the name says it all. Suck in your abdominal muscles and hold them tight for five to ten seconds. It should hurt a little if you are working them.
- The "belly dancer." Just like belly dancers, you can strengthen your stomach muscles. Do this by tightening or sucking those muscles inward, then letting them out rapidly and repeatedly. When I do this exercise, I imagine that an appreciative audience is stuffing dollar bills in my belt. Better yet, do it while J'arming (jogging with the arms). See *J'ARM for the Health of It* (CompCare Publishers).

Caring for your back

Warning signs that your back needs attention

If the following scenario seems to describe you or someone you know, pay close attention. Your body is delivering warning signs. These signs are Mother Nature's kind way of saying "do something before it's too late."

Think of the people who say, "My back always goes out once or twice a year." Generally, these are people who don't like to sit for any length of time. They don't like plane rides, attending theaters, or sitting in church. When these people stand up after sitting, they feel stiff and tight in the low back. Often they'll stand up slowly, holding the low back as they do.

These people tell me that when they exercise or walk, their low back feels better. As a matter of fact, they get up and walk every half-hour or so to keep their low back from hurting.

People who have these episodic low back pains often sleep on their sides. Seldom do they sleep on their stomachs. Yet the hours they spend sleeping on the side are merely adding to their misery, even though these people are seldom aware of the fact. All they know is: "When I wake , I ache."

These people tend to work at sedentary jobs, bending over a counter or desk all day long. Working at a computer terminal is a common occupation for people with this problem. In addition, truck drivers, assembly line workers, mechanics, and people in similar jobs spend much of their work time in the forward bent-over position. In other words, they frequently slouch forward.

Even the homemaker is not safe from episodic back pain. She (and in many cases, he) is bending—bending over the sink, bending over the beds, bending over the ironing board, bending over cribs and over the stove. Everything this group of pain sufferers does bends them forward. These are people who rarely have a chance or take the opportunity to arch their backs. Consequently, their posture is poor.

And of course, they sleep on their sides in the "fetal" position because they have been lead to believe that stomach sleeping is "bad." This side, curled-up position just adds to their poor posture problem.

What happens as a result of such poor posture? Often these people develop a bulging disc in the low back. While this bulging disc does not always give sharp pain, it can frequently give a sensation of stiffness. If the disc bulges a great deal, it can touch a nerve, or "live wire." This leads to radiating leg pain or muscle spasm. Or, the wall of the disc can have a small crack. Through that crack can spill some of the soluble disc chemicals (phospho-lipase A-2).

Studies have shown that in our population, a bulging disc is very common, particularly in those over age thirty. If CAT scans were done routinely on everyone over age fifty, a full 50 percent would show a bulging disc, even when back pain is not present. Bulging discs are common, and the amount of bulge is not static but constantly changing.

Why discs move around

Disc material is a sort of gelatinous substance much like silly putty or toothpaste. It acts as a kind of padding between the bony vertebrae.

This material is contained within a compartment that we can compare to a toothpaste tube. When we are young the disc material is almost a liquid; it's the consistency of soft butter. As we reach our thirties the disc material becomes harder, more like the consistency of toothpaste. In our forties it becomes even harder—like toothpaste when someone has forgotten to put the cap back on the tube. During our fifties it hardens into a soft putty, and into the sixties it can be a hard putty. Eventually it becomes like cement and nearly immovable.

Because disc material moves more easily in the

younger ages, disc problems are more prevalent in people in their thirties and forties and begin to occur less frequently as the population reaches their sixth and seventh decades. Back pain in the sixties and beyond, I feel, is often caused more by tight tissues than it is by disc degeneration or damaged bone. (However, a condition called spinal stenosis is due to abnormal bone impingement on the spinal cord or the nerves of the lower back. These are often amenable to surgery.)

For several reasons, the walls of the container that holds the disc material in place often become weakened or cracked. If the wall is weakened but remains intact, the disc material can bulge or herniate. But if the walls of the disc container crack, then some of the disc material can spill outside of the container. When the crack is small, only soluble, tissue-irritating toxic chemicals can escape.

If the crack becomes a tear in the wall of the disc, then the more solid disc material (along with the toxic soluble chemicals) can escape. This is called an extruded disc. The extruded disc is obviously a much more significant problem than is a herniated disc or a "toxic chemical spill" through a small crack. An extruded disc is difficult or impossible to return to the disc "container." Fortunately, extruded disc material tends to shrink with time.

To understand this, think again about the nature of that disc material. The viscous (liquid-like) disc material can be made to move back and forth within the contained disc space. It can be pushed from one end of its tube (container) to the other end. Picture a tube of toothpaste. If you push on one end, all of the toothpaste goes to the other end. And the same is true if you push on the other side. It can be moved back and forth.

Likewise, if disc material moves too far toward the back, it can cause a bulge. If that bulge touches a nerve, severe pain can result. This condition can frequently be improved by moving the disc material further forward, by returning the disc material toward its normal position or "squeezing on the toothpaste tube to relocate the toothpaste."

When the "tube" that contains the disc material ruptures, this is analogous to the seam of the toothpaste tube tearing open or the cap popping off. At this point it is difficult to get the material to return to the tube.

Often the tube has only bulged or herniated, and the container's lining is weakened but still intact. In that case, the disc material can frequently be moved back into its proper position and the bulge or hernia reduced. How? Through exercise (often a back-arching exercise) and good sitting posture—again, by aligning the ear and the rear.

Most people, before they have an acute attack of severe back discomfort, know that there is something "wrong" with their low back. Often the back is feeling stiffer than usual. This feeling of stiffness is a sign that the disc is bulging more than usual and that it is getting dangerously close to hitting one of the nerves. Or the stiffness may develop because a tiny crack has occurred in the bulging disc wall, allowing a small amount of toxic tissue chemical to seep out and irritate the back tissues.

At this stage a small amount of additional bulge could occur with a very slight movement, such as picking up a paper from the floor. This little added bulge could contact the nerves and become the "straw that broke the camel's back."

Obviously, the time to move the disc forward to a more normal position is in the early stages of bulging. By repositioning the disc material or keeping it in position with posture and proper lifting skills, we can avoid many low back problems.

A short history of back arching
I feel the leading cause of bulging discs is the constant backward pressure on the disc caused by a slouched sitting

posture. Related to this is the regrettably common belief that we should not arch the back. However, the way to get a bulging disc to return to its proper place is actually to arch the back.

When I first tell people that they must arch their backs, many of them think they've heard me wrong. "Unheard of!" they say. Like them, you've probably been told for years by "conventional medical wisdom" not to arch your back and not to sleep on the stomach. So my instruction to arch takes them by surprise.

"What? What do you want me to do, Doctor?"

"Arch, backwards," I say.

At this point, I know many wonder to themselves, "What kind of a doctor is this?" Many times these people leave my office in a state of puzzlement. Soon they telephone to tell me that a relative or friend is sure they shouldn't arch the back. I reassure them that, yes, I do want them to follow a back-arching program.

For some time now, we've lived with two detrimental messages about back care: Don't arch your back, and don't sleep on your stomach. Thirty to forty years ago, however, popular opinion was just the opposite: it was common for physicians to recommend back arching. Then American physicians broke rank and began advising against arching the back. In fact, they started prescribing a set of movements known as the Williams exercises for most back pain. These exercises focused on strengthening the stomach and front body muscles, as well as flattening the arch in the low back.

Meanwhile, physicians in Great Britain kept encouraging people to arch their backs. It's commonly felt that this significantly accounts for the lower incidence of back problems in that country.

In America today our thinking is changing. During the last five years, many in the medical community— particularly those who deal with back problems—have come to accept the arching exercises used by physicians and physical therapists in New Zealand, Australia, and England. Current research shows that arching the back is important and beneficial in treating many back conditions.

Please keep these ideas in perspective. I recommend specific arching exercises to about 90 percent of the back-pain patients I see. (These are commonly referred to by physicians as the McKenzie exercises.) Even so, there are still uses for the Williams exercises, and there are also cases where back arching is not recommended.

If you are doing the Williams exercises and they are helping, then by all means continue. If such exercises are yielding no improvement, or merely partial improvement, then you may want to try back-arching exercises. These arching exercises can be done alone, apart from other exercise. When you're doing them as part of a larger exercise routine, then do the arching exercises last.

If your physician has told you not to arch your back, I hesitate to contradict him/her. And if your back hurts more after arching exercises, or if there is any indication of pain going into your legs, then stop the arching exercises. Consult a physician or physical therapist for specific exercise suggestions.

The benefits of back arching

Arching the back has three main benefits:

- It helps move a bulging disc back into position. When you arch your back, you are in effect compressing the swollen end of the "toothpaste tube" and driving the bulge back where it belongs. It helps to envision this while you are doing the arching exercise. Think of moving the disc material toward your belly button. Really arch your back to drive the disc forward and reduce the posterior bulge.
- Back-arching stretches the stiff muscles and other soft tissues, allowing for greater ease when assuming

a proper posture. Stretched tissue also allows for greater all-around flexibility.

■ Back-arching movement also aids circulation and nutrition to the back tissues. When doing a back-arching exercise (or any back exercise for that matter), you compensate for the naturally poor circulation in the low back. A poor blood supply exists in and around back tissues because there are relatively few small blood vessels and capillaries. There is, however, good, nutritious extra cellular fluid present. You can move or "pump" this fluid around by keeping your low back mobile.

This extra cellular fluid should not be allowed to sit stagnant. By doing any low back movement, particularly back-arching exercise, you create a pumping effect that keeps the tissue fluids moving. This delivers oxygen and nutrients to the back tissue. Movement also enhances vascular circulation.

Equally important is another fact. When you increase circulation and move these tissue fluids, they wash out metabolic waste products and soluble toxic "spills" that escape through cracks in the disc wall. We can compare a cracked disk to a cracked drum containing toxic waste in a stagnant marsh. If there is no water movement, the toxins concentrate around the barrel. But when a heavy rain comes, the ground water and the marsh water dilute or wash away the offensive chemical. In a similar way, arching your low back helps to wash away chemical irritants.

Get back your youthful back

Many times I'll have patients do a back-arching exercise in my office, and I'll ask them when they are doing it: "Does it hurt?" Often they'll say yes.

"Good," I'll reply. "It's supposed to hurt a little. The reason you're having back problems is that you haven't exercised your back by arching it in a long time. The tissues that were supple when you were young are now tight and pulling you forward. Also, the muscles that hold your back up straight have become weak and frail from underuse and elongation. You need to move those muscles and restore that natural, youthful arch again in your back. You need to regenerate that degenerated back."

Many of us have seen the ads in women's magazines picturing an older woman stooped forward with "osteoporosis." Often these ads are pitching calcium supplements made from some expensive or exotic source, such as ground-up seashells from Tahiti. I do recommend that women of all ages and men over forty take calcium supplements (unless they have medical reasons not to do so). But I recommend they take it in the form of an antacid tablet that contains calcium. This provides a less expensive and equally effective form of calcium.

Back to the woman in the ad. Her "bent out of shape," little old lady (LOL) posture problem is not due to osteoporosis. Rather, her problem is due to the lifelong habit of terrible posture. Chances are she hasn't arched backward in years. We can avoid this posture by taking action now. Most of the people I see with this poor LOL posture can still improve.

Remember, as a teenager, how easily you could arch backwards? Things may have changed a bit for you since then. Good news: You can regain some of your youthful suppleness. How? By working a back-arching exercise into your life several times a day. I recommend doing this exercise two to four times daily for thirty seconds. That's just two minutes each day.

And, yes, it's okay to sleep on your stomach if that is comfortable for you. Doing so may even improve the archability of your back. I feel that sleeping on your side in the semi-fetal position can just worsen the problems caused by a poor sitting posture. By sleeping on your stomach (if and when it's comfortable) and looking for opportunities to arch your back, you will be working to regain youthful back flexibility.

Walking is a great exercise that in some ways simulates back-arching exercises. As you walk, the arch in your low back is emphasized, particularly if you concentrate on holding your head up high and keeping the "ear and the rear" lined up. Swimming is recommended for the same reason.

A safe position for cooling down

Remember that disc material is a soft, gelatinous, semi-fluid type material and, like most similar material, it changes in consistency with variations in temperature. When it is cold this material gets thicker and more difficult to move. When it is warm it moves much more easily. This is true, to various degrees (no pun intended), of all body tissues.

After exercising, many people put themselves into cool-down positions with the back slouched forward. As they do so, the warmed-up, more mobile disc material bulges and protrudes toward the rear—in the direction of the vulnerable spinal nerves. As these people sit, they cool down, and as they cool they harden into an unhealthy posture.

Look at the people who sit in a lounge chair after exercising, with their feet up on a hassock. Or, take the people who get into a typical "jock" position (see Figure 7) after exercising—sitting slouched forward on a bench with a towel draped over the neck. Their fascia, ligaments, and discs will cool down in that position too. Without meaning to, these people are setting up the conditions for poor posture and back pain.

A common wintertime scenario I see in Minnesota is the patient who works out at the health club or gym. After a "heated game," this person hurriedly takes a hot shower, rushes out into the cold, gets into a cold car, and drives twenty miles in an "over the steering wheel, " rounded-forward, slouched position—literally freezing the body tissues into the LOL/LOM posture.

Therefore, the best time to assume a good posture is when the "juices are flowing" just after exercise—before the cool-down period allows them to harden. As you cool down after "heated" exercise, try this: read a book while lying on your belly, propping your body up on your elbows. You can also sit or stand with a posture that aligns the "ear with the rear." These are excellent positions for cooling down because they arch the back. They allow the warmed tissue to cool in a stretched state and the warm, fluid disc material to gel in a healthful position.

Try this thirty-second back-arching exercise

Whenever you're feeling stiffness or back pain, do the following exercise three to four times a day in the "push-up" position.

- Lie on your stomach on the floor. Place your hands palm down in front of your shoulders. Push up, keeping your entire body from your hips down pressed firmly on the floor. Concentrate on arching the lower back. Then gently lower yourself to the floor.

  Do ten arch-ups. During the last three, extend the arms fully to their rigid position during the arch. Arch as much as possible and hold each of the last three arches for a count of 10.

- This whole sequence should take thirty to forty seconds.

- Although it's not as effective, you can also do this exercise while standing. Stand tall with your hands on your hips. (If necessary, put your hands on a stable chair or a table for support.) Arch backwards and then come back to a tall, standing position. Do ten back arches, really stretching on each of the last three and holding them for a count of 10.

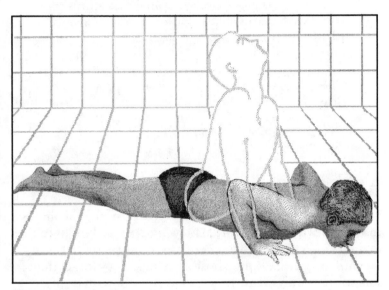

Figure 42   Arch-up exercise

Cautions: When doing the exercise while standing, proceed slowly and stop if you have any signs of dizziness. Make sure that any support is sturdy and that your feet are firmly anchored to the floor.

If the arching exercise hurts a little (up to a 3 on a 0–10 pain scale) while you are doing it, that's a good pain. It means your back needed a good stretching. However, if it hurts after you've finished, then don't continue. And if you feel any pains radiating in the buttocks or shooting down your legs, stop the exercise.

People over age sixty are advised against doing this exercise unless their physician approves. Also, people with a diagnosis of spinal stenosis should not do the exercise. (Note: People with spinal stenosis often get more—not less—back pain when they walk.)

Those who have abnormal spinal curvatures such as scoliosis, or exaggerated lumbar arch—"sway back"—or those with the diagnosis of spondylolisthesis should not do the arching exercises.

People to whom these disclaimers apply need to discuss their pains with a physician. Your physician or therapist may direct you to modify the arching exercise or prescribe additional exercises.

Allowing yourself some pain

I see so many people with pain who give up doing the things that they love to do. Too often they unnecessarily allow pain to interfere with their lives. Because certain activities bring on pain, they cease doing those activities. They forget that this strategy only creates a negative cycle, or pain trap: It hurts when I move, so I stop moving. But when I stop moving, it hurts even more, and I move even less. In the long run, this worsens pain levels, and then the pain becomes both physical and emotional. Their bodies stiffen up. They get uptight—literally. They lose out on the healthy pleasures of life.

I invite all who have pain as a result of a musculoskeletal dysfunction to join the living again. Become more active and alive. It is possible. It won't happen overnight. But by changing your lifestyle and refusing to center your life on pain, you can make it happen. You can be more alive tomorrow than you are today, and even more alive the next day than you will be tomorrow. Just allow yourself to let go of the focus on pain.

In general, we've been taught that pain is bad. Even some physicians say so. Consequently, some prescribe many different kinds of medication to mask pain, often at the patient's insistence. This is shortsighted. Some pain is not only good but necessary. Without it, we stay trapped in a low activity level. "No pain, no gain" is in fact true.

Recently I saw a woman who had been in a car accident. In the accident, a couple of her ribs were broken. This is an extremely painful injury, as anyone who has broken a rib will tell you. She came into my office hunched, stiff, and sore. She was still hurting from the accident, which occurred four months earlier.

Everything this woman did favored the area of her sore healed ribs. When she sat, she sat crooked. When she walked, she walked bent over. When she tried to straighten up, she simply couldn't do so. It hurt too much.

This woman's lack of activity following the accident allowed the injured muscles and other tissues around her broken ribs to become weak, tight, and shortened from underuse. She developed tight scar tissue around the breaks. When she attempted to straighten up, she pulled on all this tight scar and other tissues. That pulling hurt. She was convinced that all pain is harmful. So, she fell into a pattern of avoiding pain. In short, she stopped moving.

In actuality, permitting or even encouraging some pain by stretching her tight scar and other tissues is the best thing she could have done. By allowing herself some pain, she could have improved.

Looking at your own experience of pain

When we talk about allowing some pain in your life, we come quickly to a crucial question: How do I evaluate and tolerate pain?

Everyone has a personal pain scale. Think of that scale as going from 0 to 10. A 9 on one person's scale may be a 3 to someone else. The same degree of injury feels agonizing to some but causes only a minor irritation to others. This makes it important for each of us to recognize our personal pain reality—our own high or low pain tolerance.

It's at level 3 that most of us start to exhibit pain—for example, we start to limp with foot or ankle pain. When training, stretching, or exercising, make it your goal to keep your pain level around 3.

Pain and the brain

The mind plays an essential role in interpreting painful stimuli. Our reaction to such stimuli varies widely from situation to situation. While we do not create pain in the mind, our minds often determine the severity of discomfort. I never tell people that their pain is all in the head. But often I do tell them that the "volume control" for their pain may be largely in the head. With apologies to Lerner and Loewe: "The reign of pain is mainly in the brain."

The point of drawing a connection between pain on the one hand and stress, attitudes, or feelings on the other is not to feel guilty about "choosing" illness. Rather, we merely want to be aware of the mental dimension in health. Instead of blaming yourself for the stress and illness in your life, seek to understand and accept the total process of pain without judgment. Then, focus on moving forward—on relieving pain and preventing illness. Use all the strategies at your disposal, including a modification in feeling and attitude. Being confident that you will get over much or all of your pain speeds up the process. Just as in driving a car. When you put yourself behind the (pain) wheel, you have more control, confidence, and a better idea of "where you're going" and how you're going to get there.

Don't dwell on the changes you have to make in your habits. The word *change* is negative and implies that you have been doing something wrong. Rather, think positively. Concentrate on growing, building new habits, and becoming better. See yourself well. Develop a pos"I"tive "I"mage of the person you can be. And bel"I"eve it will happen!

Living with pain

Living without pain isn't what we are after. Sometimes living with pain is unavoidable. Our goal is to reduce the negative, crippling grip of pain that holds back some of its victims.

Some people, after starting an exercise program, will come into my office and tell me that their pain has not changed since the last time I saw them. I tell them that while the pain may be the same, it's time to look at their activity levels. In many cases these people previously stopped walking, biking, or working out. Now they are doing these activities again. In addition, they're often attending more social activities—parties, church functions, civic and sporting events. Indeed, they are improving. These people are continuing to grade themselves by their pain. I'm grading them instead by their activity and connection to other people.

These people often find that the severity of their pain may continue at the same level, even as they become more active. But again, it's unrealistic to focus only on eliminating pain. People may feel pain as long as their physical condition improves, especially if they were out of shape to begin with. Their pain might not diminish significantly until they once again stretch and strengthen their bodies, and until their social and physical activities allow them to replace negative thinking with pos"I"tive thinking.

Good pains and bad pains

There is no escaping it. We are all going to experience pain at various points in our lives. Pains are Mother Nature's message that we should be doing something differently (often more, not less) in our lives. We're wise to heed these messages.

For instance, when we sit for too long in one position, we begin to get uncomfortable. Pressure on one site of the body causes a reduction in blood supply, depriving that area of nutrition and oxygen, and allowing toxins to build up. So we shift our position automatically to relieve this situation. When our fingers touch something hot, we feel pain and—as airline pilots say—we make a "mid-flight correction": we change course and move the fingers. From this perspective, pain is a blessing. There really are good pains as well as bad pains.

When it comes to stretching and building muscles, we purposefully inflict some pain on ourselves—good pain. Keeping the body in good biomechanical working condition will help condition other systems, such as the cardiovascular system. This has a profound impact on all other organ systems of the body.

Because the word *pain* has such a negative connotation in our society, we could be better off thinking of good pain as discomfort. Learning the difference between good pain and bad pain is fundamental. By allowing some good pains (discomfort), you are actually helping to prevent or lessen some of the bad pains.

More about bad pains

Yes, there most definitely are bad pains. What are they? In general, bad pains are those that come at the beginning of a movement and do not improve as the activity continues. For example, if you try to walk on a broken bone in your foot, you will feel sharp pains the moment you step down. Each succeeding step will feel as painful or even worse. In contrast, inflammatory conditions or tight tissue pulls will be painful with initial movement but improve with continuing activity.

Remember that what we're talking about here is pain that begins with a specific, limited motion. Any pain that you feel at the beginning of a total program of physical fitness—such as regular walking or jogging—is not necessarily bad pain. In fact, stretching and exercising formerly inactive muscles may result in a short-lived, good pain that confirms your positive choice of a more active lifestyle.

After sitting in one position for a while, people with an inflammatory condition or tight tissues will feel stiff when they begin to move. In these cases, their joint fluids and other body tissues have cooled and thickened. Just as a car's lubricant on a cold morning needs to be warmed up, people with stiffness also need to get their bodies warmed up. Pain will be felt when they initially stand up and start moving.

For these people, a "beginning pain" is fine. In most other situations, however, beginning pains should be considered bad pains.

Another bad pain is pain that lingers after completing an activity. Pain you feel while stretching is good pain. This is stretching discomfort. Once you have stopped exercising, the discomfort should be minor, such as getting a little stiff or sore with some movements. If your pain persists, if it increases to more than a 3 on a scale of 0 to 10, or if it cannot be lessened by movement, then stop exercising. Consult your physician.

If while doing any activity you feel pains shooting down your legs or into your buttocks, those can also be bad pains. In these cases you should stop exercising immediately. These pains may indicate nerve pinching. Any chest pain is potentially dangerous. Discuss these with your physician.

Using the pain scale

Good pains include the discomfort experienced at the end of a stretch or movement. It is these ending pains that stretch the "rubber bands" out. However, even these good pains should not be overdone.

I've already referred to a pain scale going from 0 to 10, and now I'd like to explain this in more detail. By using this concept it is possible to monitor and control your own pain levels. Even though this scale is totally subjective, you'll find it practical.

Think of 0 as being no pain. A 10 is hair pulling, horrible, screaming pain. I tell my patients that I don't want them to have anything over a 4 pain. However, I do encourage you to have 1, 2, or 3 pains.

When you stretch and start to experience discomfort at the end of your stretch, this is one of the good pains. When you get into a 2 or 3 pain, I want you to try to sneak over into a 4 pain for a just a little bit. Then you can relax. It's this pushing yourself to allow a 4 pain that eventually helps decrease your general pain level.

Healing the emotional side of pain

When I started caring for patients over thirty-five years ago, physicians and patients spoke little about the mental components of pain. At that time, we judged the mind and the body to be separate entities. Fortunately we have matured with the knowledge that the mind and body are one. What we think and feel affects the structures of the body, and the biomechanical functions of the body affect the mind. In short, pains influence feelings and feelings influence pains.

Why is this still so difficult for many to accept? No doubt because for centuries our medical and religious teachings preached the duality of mind and body. Let's get real and recognize our oneness and totality of mind and body.

This perspective is especially useful when it comes to healing the emotional side of physical pain. Some pains are more emotionally disabling than physically disabling. Fortunately, just as we can stretch out and relax our physical "rubber bands," we can do the same with the emotional scars of an injury.

I know this directly, because I've spent a lifetime stretching my emotional and physical scars. When I was eighteen months old, I pulled a pot of boiling sugar water off a stove. My hands and face were severely burned. After months of healing, these third-degree burns resulted in tight, unattractive scars on my chin, neck, chest, and hands. And the accident left deep, if unseen, scars of the psyche as well.

During my early adolescent years—years when people are highly aware of their bodies—I found it difficult to look in the mirror. While attending junior high, I needed six separate plastic surgery procedures and skin grafting to remove and release some of the tight scar tissue. And for years prior to that surgery, I had to live with disfigurement to my left hand and the left side of my face and neck.

Throughout those years it was hard for me to accept that I didn't look "normal." Kids can be cruel to others who aren't perfect, and I knew from an early time that I was not perfect. I found myself walking with my good side facing people. I always entered doors with a strategy thought out completely. If I went to a public gathering such as a sporting event, I would enter so that my "good side" was toward the audience. I'd sit on the left side of the room so fewer people in the group could see my left side. I was becoming a "one-sided" half-person. Fortunately I did not try to hide my right side. If only—I often thought—if only I could just be all right.

Upon returning to school after some of my first surgical procedures, I experienced an important event—one that started healing some of my emotional scars. At that time I had a science teacher, Ms. Magner, who helped me realize how much I'd been limiting myself. I went to Ms. Magner to explain why I'd been away—not an easy thing to do, because I was so sensitive about the surgery that I didn't even like talking about it. She looked at me and said, "Surgery on the neck and face? What a surprise! Here you've been in my class all year and I never noticed that you had any scars."

Whether she did or didn't notice, this was the best thing she could have ever said. I realized that I had been so consumed by my painful feeling of "ugliness" that I was carrying around needless emotional scars—scars that prevented me from fully participating in life.

After that mental boost, I became very active in school. I simply forgot that I wasn't perfect. My reasoning was this: I'm becoming popular despite my mental scars. So why not stretch more? Why not become active in sports, drama, and student government? It worked. I was starting to think positively—pretty good for a guy who wasn't "all right."

At that impressionable stage I started reading a lot of self-help books. Dale Carnegie's *How To Win Friends and Influence People* became one of the important books in my life. I learned how other people would become interested in me if, instead of focusing on my problems and pains, I got interested in them. I learned from Carnegie that I'd been given "lemons"—my scars of body and mind—and that I could make lemonade out of them. In other words, I've learned to take what might be a disadvantage and turn it around to my advantage. You can do the same.

Having experienced many surgeries, pain, and physical and mental scarring, I believe, has made me a more sensitive physician. I know firsthand how an injury can change your life—even years after the original event. In fact, shortly after completing a surgical residency at the Mayo Clinic, the scars on my hand began to cause problems. This forced me to give up surgery. My hands simply couldn't hold up in surgical rubber gloves for hours. In addition, the hand scars started to break down and refused to heal. More skin grafting, this time of the left hand, was necessary. Any idea of continuing a surgical practice for another twenty to thirty years was simply impractical.

At the time this felt like the end of the world. Actually it was the beginning of new opportunities: an opportunity to work for Johnson and Johnson and 3M as associate director of clinical research; an opportunity to become active and board-certified in emergency medicine; an opportunity to study pain treatment and mobilization techniques; an opportunity to join the highly regarded Park Nicollet Medical Center in Minneapolis. This wonderful group of colleagues gave me the opportunity to develop speaking and educational skills as medical director of SHAPE, a health education program of Park Nicollet Medical Foundation. SHAPE's mission is to teach nonmedical audiences the benefits of knowledgeable self-care and healthy lifestyles. Most importantly, I've had an opportunity to write this book and share *Fold and Hold* with you.

I say all this not to shine a light on myself, but to illustrate one point: Pain, disfigurement, and disappointment do not have to stop you. Instead, if you do a "mid-flight correction" in your thinking and behavior, these circumstances can lead you to possibilities beyond imagination. When we live with this sense of possibility, we not only uncover a secret of pain control—we learn about how to live.

My wish is that all your pains—whether of the body or mind—become good pains in this larger sense. And may *Fold and Hold* be the first step on that path for you.

About the author

Dale L. Anderson, M.D., has been a physician for thirty-three years and has practiced as a family doctor, a board certified surgeon, and a board certified emergency physician. His current clinical practice is in the Biomechanics Clinic of the Orthopedic Department of Park Nicollet Medical Center in Minneapolis—the country's fifth largest multispecialty clinic. He is on the staff of Methodist Hospital in Minneapolis, and is a clinical assistant professor at the University of Minnesota Medical School.

Dr. Anderson, a member of the National Speakers Association and one of America's leading health "edu-tainers," conducts seminars nationally through his own speaking company, J'Arm, Inc. His book, *J'Arm for the Health of It*, also published by CompCare Publishers, is about "jogging with the arms" in a "conducting" movement and other easy things to do to keep fit, feel better, and raise your endorphin level. An audio tape, *J'Arm for the Health of It*, is also available from CompCare.

About the illustrations

The illustrations in this book are the result of a image-creating partnership between artist, Al Hage, and his Amiga computer, which is video-interactive. Video is used to capture actions, such as the *Fold and Hold* procedures in this book, and these "motion pictures" can be introduced directly into the computer, frame by frame. With the image on the computer screen, shapes and tones are modified, unwanted sections eliminated, and clips from other frames are imported and positioned. This amounts to adding, subtracting, moving, and retouching. Traditionally, making changes on a finished drawing can be very time-consuming and limiting. In computer graphics, the illustrations need never be considered "finished." They are, says Hage, more process than product.

The illustrations here, uniform in tone and in selective detail, are published as "line art" with the text. The artist, appropriately, signs the drawings used in this technique "AlandAmiga."